Praise for *Oh Mama*

Kathy Fray is a global thought leader on integrative maternity healthcare. This introductory overview guide is a pioneering breakthrough – right out there on the cutting-edge of holistic maternal/neonatal wellness. A copy needs to be in the back pocket of every midwife and obstetrician.

ROBBIE DAVIS-FLOYD, PhD, Texas, USA
World-renowned Medical Anthropologist, Childbirth/Midwifery/
Obstetrics Researcher and Speaker

Such an eye-opening book that holds so much potential for maternity care! It is a gentle reminder of the array of possibilities we can seek, yet not so many people know about!

NOUR ZAKI, Ph.D., Egypt
Pre/Peri/Post-natal Therapist and Assistant Professor at American
University Cairo

On a sick planet, where nature is being destroyed in the name of a fantasy of 'progress', our medical systems are also in the ICU. The radical medical invasion of our body through countless drugs – from the first minutes of life until the moment of death – has produced a society that only believes in healthcare when it comes from the outside, through the bombardment of technology to which we all are subjected. Now is the time to question the old paradigm of medicine. This book by Kathy Fray proposes a renewal in health thinking. Her invitation to this journey through various healing models is a balm for everyone who wants to learn safe ways to resuscitate maternity healthcare through new/old models of healing.

RICARDO H JONES, MD, Brazil
Obstetrician, Homeopath, Author, International Lecturer

Any time an experienced practitioner can bring forward the wisdom of their knowledge, is a beneficial time for all connected to that field.

With 'Oh Mama' Kathy uses her extensive experience as a case-loading midwife as well as her desire to traverse the turbidity that exists in regards to Natural Medicine in pregnancy, and begins a much needed discussion to bring clarity to the possibilities and options available to couples and practitioners alike, when it comes to Natural and Integrative Maternity Care.

WINTON TERRY. Australia
Acupuncturist, Natural Birth Specialist, Former BSc TCM Ob/Gyn Unit
Coordinator for Victoria University of Tech

Kathy has done it again – this is a brilliant, forthright and practical guide. We are reminded of the atrocious state of health and wellbeing in the world. It is time for integrative maternity healthcare providers to join force and collaborate for more successful and natural birth journeys and outcomes. This book is aimed as a guide for all birth practitioners to help support, nurture and empower mothers along their pregnancy journey. As a mother and chiropractor who is passionate about working with women perinatally, this is a must read for all birth practitioners. Thank you, Kathy for your passion, vision and determination to make holistic maternal and neonatal wellness the norm.

KATIE PRITCHARD, New Zealand
Advanced Chiropractor Practitioner

I love this latest book from Kathy Fray that combines her years of midwifery experience with a much-needed overview of holistic approaches to the childbirth process and maternity journey. In a world where we have become so dependent on prescription medications and surgical interventions, Kathy's point of view is a breath of fresh air.

This book is a 'must have' for any mother-to-be and Birth

Practitioner looking to forego what has become 'routine' medical interventions in lieu of healthier, more holistic management care-plans.

Jocelyn M. Wood, M.A. CCC-SLP, New York USA
Bilingual Speech Language Pathologist

In her new book Kathy Fray delivers incredible gold for practitioners and mothers alike. Knowing how to holistically care for the mother during conception and pregnancy is such a minefield, even more so as the maternity process has become so radically medicalized over the past 80 years. Armed with this guide, we can select or recommend tested support options that sit within integrity with life, with nature, and protect and restore our womb's precious homeostasis ... Introducing the different modalities so beautifully and succinctly in plain English can help the parents (-to be) as much as the practitioners, well beyond pregnancy and birth. A must-have resource. I don't know how we could live without it!

NATHALIE BELLE-LARANT, New Zealand
Author, Speaker, Transformational Fertility Coach, Matrescence Alchemist and Soul Midwife

Oh Mama ... Perinatal Integrative Healthcare

Oh Mama ...

Perinatal Integrative Healthcare

Birth Practitioner Guide to Holistic Maternal/Neonatal Wellness

KATHY FRAY

Published by MotherWise

Contact: www.MothersWise.com

A catalogue record for this book is available from the National Library of New Zealand.

DISCLAIMER

The purpose of the information presented in this book is to protect, promote and support normal birth by reducing unnecessary interventions. However, this guide should never substitute for advice from medical clinicians, particularly obstetric physicians. Medical 'best practice' still applies regarding maternal/neonatal healthcare matters, especially diagnosis and treatment management plans for complex complications.

This is not a medical textbook. It is an introductory overview of complementary/alternative natural therapeutic modalities and practitioner treatment remedies which may partially, or fully, positively affect maternity health and wellness to assist to keep things normal. Birth Practitioners incorporating such perinatal integrative medicine into their practices should undertake recognised educational training in such therapies or refer their clients to qualified practitioners.

Oh Mama ... is dedicated to all the forthright, rebellious, non-conforming, revolutionary, dissident mavericks on this planet, who routinely live their lives as radical, innovative, pioneering, unconventional, cutting-edge leaders; who make tangible differences, creating innovative changes for transformative impact.

Being a tall poppy ain't the easy route to choose, so I toast you, friends.

I toast us all!

Contents

The Antepartum (Pregnancy)

The Intrapartum (Childbirth)

The Postpartum (First Six Weeks Postnatal)

Author's Note

It is no measure of health to be well adjusted to a profoundly sick society.

Jiddu Krishnamurti, Indian philosopher (1895–1986)

This book is no minor "accidental" occurrence.

From my perspective as the writer, it is the culmination of a series of serendipitous events, spanning three decades: resulting in a sense of author's karmic destiny, with the "meant-to-be" sensation occurring at a visceral level.

From your perspective as the reader, it is completely logical to ask a *"Who the heck is Kathy Fray?"* question as to why the heck I'm writing this holistic birth practitioner's guide to maternity wellness (aka *Perinatal Integrative Healthcare*). That's a good question. And to be honest, sometimes when the tall poppy syndrome is being especially brutal, I can find myself asking the same question. But most of the time I know *exactly* why this topic has become my compelled passion: It's simply purpose ... fate ... vocation ... dharma.

In an effort to avoid a verbose prologue, here is a brief summary of my integrative medicine personal and professional journey that has brought you and I (reader and writer) to this moment ...

My fascination for general integrative medicine began at 19 years of age when I experienced an "astonishing" cure through acupuncture for recurrent abdominal pain ... then in my mid-20s I experienced a "wondrous" cure through reiki for another chronic condition ... then aged 30 I experienced an "incredible" cure through herbalism for ongoing infertility

... then in my early–mid-30s I experienced multiple mind-blowing cures through homeopathy for our young children's unwellnesses ... and by then I was hooked! Hook, line and sinker – addicted to the actual reality that complementary therapies and alternative modalities are *no* pseudo-science (as so often touted by the ignorant and belligerent). Such ancient and modern, traditional and progressive healing treatments can routinely be amazing, wonderful, astounding, phenomenal, marvellous, extraordinary, and scientifically inexplicable.

In the early 2000s, in my late 30s, now with a truck-load of maternity and IM (integrative medicine) first-hand experience, I began writing about integrative maternity healthcare with my first book, *Oh Baby ... Birth, Babies & Motherhood Uncensored*, which has been a best-seller for publishers Penguin Random House ever since.

In 2005, aged 40, I knew it was time to broaden my maternity knowledge academically, and so commenced a formal degree in midwifery.

Five years later, in 2010, while working as a case-loading 24/7 on-call midwife (for nearly the next decade, catching *hundreds* of babies), my second book was published in North America, *Oh Grow Up: Toddlers to Preteens Decoded*, complete with its encyclopaedic-style chapters on integrative medicine for children.

In 2015, as recipient of a small seed-money grant, I founded the SOMCANZ (Symposium of Maternity Carers Australia & New Zealand) inaugural conference on integrative maternity healthcare, which was a huge success – beyond my wildest expectations.

Over the following years, SOMCANZ collaborated with AIMA (Australasian Integrative Medicine Association) as their 'perinatal division'. This was a wonderful professional alliance, however with our database growing by thousands internationally, five things became obvious:

- It was time to rename from a local to worldwide operation: IIMHCO (International Integrative Maternity HealthCare Organization).
- We needed to create a regular IMHC (Integrative Maternity HealthCare) Research e-Journal for our exponentially growing mailing list.
- It was time to plan a first "global summit" on perinatal integrative medicine, titled the Maternity Natural Health Symposium.
- We needed to be "part of the solution" to narrowing the gap between academic research and expectant mothers-to-be – due to too much information known at the tertiary level, never heard about at the coalface.
- A succinct introductory overview guidebook to perinatal integrative medicine was needed for birth practitioners to feel more confident with their competence around holistic maternity healthcare. (Thus, here we now are, you and I, in this prologue.)

When I wrote my number one best-seller *Oh Baby*, I was not any kind of qualified maternity health professional. I was simply a mother, writing for other mothers (with exhaustive investigative research supported by multiple qualified specialist experts). And that, I believe, is why *Oh Baby* has been such a success: it's a practical, compassionate, grounded yet ethereal, and a "very real" non-judgmental guide, written honestly one mother to another, with a strong focus on using the natural to preserve the normal.

When I wrote my second book, *Oh Grow Up*, it was snapped-up by an American publisher but of course I was not a "qualified child psychologist". I was simply a parent, writing for other parents (once again, with exhaustive investigative research supported by multiple qualified specialist experts). And that, I also believe, is why *Oh Grow Up* is still in print: it too is a practical, compassionate, grounded yet ethereal, non-judgmental guide, written from one parent to another, introducing the concept of "wholistic triadic" parenting, with a strong focus on using the natural to uphold the normal.

When I wrote my third book, *Oh God – What the Hell Do I Tell Them?! Guide for Vaguely Spiritual Parents*, it came runner-up in prestigious body-mind-spirit book awards, even though I was not a religious or academic scholar. I was simply a work-in-progress, writing for other works-in-progress (and again, as author, being supported by multiple specialist experts). And that, I believe, is why it was award-receiving: it was simple, down-to-earth wisdom.

With writing this fourth book, *Oh Mama … Perinatal Integrative Healthcare: Birth Practitioner Guide to Holistic Maternal/Neonatal Wellness*, once again I am not a qualified naturopathic practitioner of any specific therapeutic modality. I am simply one birth practitioner, writing for other birth practitioners (obstetricians, midwives, doulas, childbirth educators), providing investigative research supported by many qualified specialist experts. And that, I believe, is why you will find this guidebook beneficial: it's real, practical, in-the-trenches wisdom.

To conclude with a little rant …

Alarmingly, our children's generation today are now the first generation ever predicted to have shorter lifespans than their parents.

Today hubby Mark and my children, all 'yadults' (young adults), have collectively been alive for well over 60 years, yet none of them yet has ever needed a course of antibiotics for a secondary infection.

I am not "anti" antibiotics. And our kids *have* been sick.

I am simply "anti" antibiotics being prescribed as the first cab off the rank.

It was luck none of our children was born prematurely or with congenital anomalies. But it is not just luck that they are this healthy. It is knowledge of what influences *wellness* that has resulted in this lack of *dis-ease*.

And nearly a quarter of a century ago, as a health-conscious wannabe, expectant parent, I knew instinctively it must *all begin in the womb*.

Love and light,

Kathy xxx

Preface

The reason one vitamin can cure so many illnesses is because a deficiency of one vitamin can cause many illnesses.

Andrew Saul, therapeutic nutritionist

If there is *one* mindset required, perhaps more than anything else, when working with integrative medicine, it is always maintaining a deep respect for pragmatic "real-world" research, new knowledge, and innovative methodologies.

Also considering the unceasing conservatives' anti-alternative rhetoric, let me add a personal observation: not liking a *person* and not liking a *person's opinion* are two completely different things. And lest we forget, when we choose not to like a person *because* of their opinion, that rigid narrow outlook is termed "small-mindedness".

When I step back in time, to when I began my university studies, this is when I began to discover fundamentally, as a burgeoning health professional, that although modern medicine talks of the body naturally seeking homeostatic equilibrium, the reality is the training of our hospital doctors focuses its teaching on *patho*physiology – not wellness.

I learned hospitals are rife with something called *nosocomial infections* – bugs that dominantly only live in hospital wards, which gives us the acronym HAI (hospital-acquired infections).

I learned that if I want to get knowledgeable about health – as opposed to being knowledgeable about dis-ease – then I need to learn these insights from the naturopathic therapeutic modalities, especially those most ancient. Because let's face it, modern scientific medicine has been correcting its incorrect advice since the beginning of its inception.

If we take the humble chicken egg as one simple example:

Thousands of years ago the chicken egg was regarded as an easy-to-hunt nutritious food source.

Then 3000 years ago the chicken and its eggs became a domesticated healthy food supply.

In the 1950s–60s, well-known advert slogans were created, like "A chicken in every pot" and "When there's an egg in the house, there's a meal in the house" (interestingly, the latter jingle was first coined by my own father, Ron Boon, as the marketing executive managing the NZ Egg Board's advertising).

In the 1970s, cholesterol research decreed *no more than three eggs a week* to avoid cardiovascular disease (a scientific announcement that devastated commercial egg farming at the time). Plus, in the 1970s movie *Rocky*, Sylvester Stallone drinks raw eggs on screen, which lit a fire under its consumption for body-builders (with nutritionists arguing there's more protein in cooked eggs, and bacteriologists warning of the potential for salmonella poisoning).

In the 1980s, nutrition guideliners set out to re-educate the public's growing scepticism around egg cholesterol being bad, and by the 1990s new nutrition guidelines stated 1.5 eggs a day equates to permissible cholesterol (and the public mused how to cut an uncooked egg in half).

In the 2000s, many countries around the world started to

remove all national weekly dietary restrictions on eggs, and by 2013 latest research headlines around the world were confirming no association whatsoever between egg consumption and cardiovascular disease.

Interesting aside: in 2016 the oldest living person on earth, Emma Morano, was crediting her longevity to eating raw eggs (and her physician publicly confirmed her cholesterol levels were excellent).

And today what is medical science's current understandings around eating chicken eggs? Well, these days we know there is actually a distinct correlation between eating eggs daily and reduced cardiovascular disease. Now the motto is "An egg a day keeps the doctor away".

Good grief.

And this is just the simplest summary of medical science's journey around *one* basic food source!

Such constant drastic revisions of medical advice makes questioning medical advice not just a reasonable thing to do, but actually an intelligently logical thing to do. Without entering the inoculation debate, it is interesting to note that for many years now, the lowest vaccination rates in Sydney, Australia have been occurring within the most affluent suburbs (no longer the lower socio-economic areas). The "God Syndrome" for doctors has disintegrated. Dr Google and Dr YouTube are having stronger influences on the tertiary-educated parents of today – and that's a *massive* swing in societal mentality away from trusting mainstream medicine.

So yes, like many of us today, we are realizing that if we want to get knowledgeable about health – as opposed to being knowledgeable about dis-ease – then we need to open our minds towards the radical and even the fringe, and certainly towards the traditional and most ancient, and without doubt towards the innovative and cutting edge.

If your child is premature, or they break a bone, or they have an anatomical abnormality – then modern paediatrics, especially surgically, can potentially save your child's life with miraculous scientific technology.

However, the fact is abundantly clear we have exponentially increasing levels of hospitals full of patients with chronic long-term coronary disease, and cancer victims begging life to consecrate them to the status of cancer survivors – all being provided healthcare that continues to feed our sick with white breads, overcooked soggy vegetables and random gelatinous desserts. How on this earth can our healthcare systems remain so nutritiously dumb?

And then of course we have Big Pharma – a juggernaut that would bankrupt instantly if a simple, natural, inexpensive cure for cancer was confirmed. We must all face the facts: there are just too many trillions of dollars tied up in Big Pharma to avoid corruption.

In the UK today, three times as many people die annually from the side effects of their prescribed medications versus the numbers who die in vehicle accidents. It's true, yet a statistic rarely talked about.

In the USA today, over six million children have been diagnosed with ADHD, equivalent to two children in every American classroom being medicated. It's talked about *in perpetuum*, but commercially it's great business.

I could write a novel on the corruption within Big Pharma!

Additional to all the *physiological* disease is the rampant *psychological* disease. Statistics show that a phenomenal quarter of our adult Western population annually are prescribed anti-depressants; including almost one-third of our working mothers – then again, the full-time stay-at-home mothers are statistically even more at risk for depression.

Today our Ritalin- and Ventolin-fed hyper-allergenic children are being cared for by their Losec- and Prozac-fed parents, and babysat by their warfarin- and insulin-fed grandparents.

We are now entire nations of overfed, undernourished, recurrently diseased, and desperately depressed people.

We must seriously question why we have become the sickliest generation ever to exist, when it's never been so possible to be healthy. And we must ask why we have become one of the saddest generations of humans ever to have roamed this Earth, when human life has never had so many labour-saving luxuries.

In the words of renowned nutrition scientist Professor Jeffrey Bland, so much of the population today is "vertically ill" – not sick enough to be lying down (horizontally ill), but certainly not *well*.

However today, as women, as parents, and as patients, we are demanding a new paradigm!

In September 2014, Emma Watson, lead actor from the eight Harry Potter movies, and UN Women Goodwill Ambassador, delivered a riveting address to the United Nations on women's rights. Adapting the speech specifically to the topic of maternity care, is so apt:

> If obstetric medicine doesn't have to control, women's naturopathic medicine won't have to be controlled. Both modern obstetrics and traditional naturopathics should feel free to be sensitive. Both obstetrics and naturopathics should feel free to be strong.
>
> It is time we all perceive all medicine on one spectrum instead of two sets of opposing ideals.
>
> I want consulting obstetricians to take up this mantel, so that their obstetric registrars can be free from birthing narrow-mindedness. But also, so that their own daughters have permission to embrace naturopathically assisted normal childbirth too, reclaiming those parts of their own intuitive Mother Nature they'd abandoned. And in doing so, become a more complete and fulfilled version of themselves.
>
> As health professionals, if we stop defining each other by what we are not, and start defining ourselves by who we are, birthing women can all be freer.

Introduction

The idea of minimum or maximum amounts of any nutrient is utterly ridiculous! We've gotten so chemically smart we're stupid.

Don Tolman, self-care wholefood activist

In 2014–2015, I was the founding director of a global inaugural conference on integrative maternity healthcare, which was a ground-breaking and revolutionary symposium, held in Auckland, New Zealand. This conference promoted a cross-discipline exchange of progressive research, innovative knowledge, enlightened experience and radical ideas; all in a medically professional and universally holistic environment of visionary open-mindedness.

Until then, maternity health specialists could convene only under their individual professional organizational umbrellas – but this symposium was, at last, a gathering for *all* maternity professionals to connect and communicate with each other. From midwives to medical herbalists, from hypnobirthers to homeopaths, from obstetricians to osteopaths, and every therapeutic discipline in between; with our collective goal being to uphold the World Health Organization mandate:

Optimal health and wellbeing are inclusive of the physical, social, psychological, emotional and spiritual dimensions of life.

At the same time, working in maternity care for the past decades, I have always yearned for the availability of an IMHC (Integrative Maternity HealthCare) guidebook that summarizes an overview of these ancient and contemporary wisdoms ... a literary place where all maternity health specialists of every therapeutic modality are convened together, contained within one succinct and user-friendly introductory handbook. And, as the old adage says, I came to the full realization "If it is to be, it is up to me". Thus, this book.

To be logical, we need to begin with definitions:

What are CAMs and T&CMs?

CAMs (complementary and alternative medicines) and T&CMs (traditional and complementary medicines) are fundamentally the "same animal" – and can roughly be divided into five sub-categories:

- Traditional medicines (e.g. homeopathy, medical herbalism, essential oils, Chinese medicine, Indian Ayurveda)
- Mind-body connections (e.g. meditation, spiritual healing, NLP [neuro-linguistic programming], music, dance)
- Biological nourishment (e.g. diet, vitamins, minerals, supplements)
- Body manipulation (e.g. chiropractic, osteopathy)
- Energy healing (e.g. reiki, qigong, pulsed electromagnetic fields).

What are HTMMs and AMMAs?

At IIMHCO we believe it is inappropriate to describe any *one* therapy of medicine as being "mainstream", "conventional" or "orthodox". The medicine that is "mainstream" for any human being (i.e. normal, ordinary, and used by the local majority) depends entirely on where you live. The medicine that is "conventional" (i.e. regular, conforming, established) depends on what the usual norm is within your cultural traditions. And the medicine that is "orthodox" (i.e. approved, accepted, standard) can only be determined by the behaviour that conforms within your local society.

Consequently, it is logical we permanently re-define treatment modalities as:

- HTMMs – holistic traditional and modern medicines (what many currently refer to as CAMs or T&CMs, which have historically focused on eliminating the *cause* of dis-ease)
- AMMAs – allopathic modern medicine alternatives (what many currently refer to as mainstream conventional medicine, which has empirically focused on reducing the *symptoms* of disease).

What is IM (integrative medicine)?

Integrative medicine (IM) is healing-oriented medicine that is holistic (i.e. takes account of the whole person). It focuses on eliminating the cause of symptoms, rather than only reducing the side effects of symptoms.

IM also emphasizes the therapeutic relationship between practitioner and patient; is informed by evidence; and potentially makes use of multiple therapies.

At its root foundation, IM incorporates the use of both HTTMs *and* AMMAs.

What is IMHC/PIM?

Integrative maternity healthcare (IMHC) is specifically the maternity healthcare division of IM (integrative medicine). Thus, IMHC can also be called PIM (perinatal integrative medicine) i.e. holistic maternal/neonatal wellness.

IMHC definition

When the medical and the holistic; the modern and the traditional; the allopathic and the naturopathic; all respect how they complement each other, to deliberately form a united revolution of cohesive evolution, to create the ultimate in *best maternity care*.

In practical terms, IMHC or PIM can be witnessed successfully operating first-hand at an IM maternity antenatal clinic, when for example all under one roof, a woman can see her customary midwife, her medical obstetrician, her traditional doula, a holistic homeopath, a naturopathic herbalist, plus other therapies such as ancient acupuncture and modern osteopathy.

Important points to note regarding this book

This is a birth practitioner's *introductory overview* to IMHC (integrative maternity healthcare). This is not a definitive textbook reference on perinatal integrative medicine.

Please *do not* use the information contained within this book to definitively treat or diagnose.

If you are not educated in any particular modality, you

---

should not be prescribing from it. Diagnostic therapies mentioned throughout this book are examples for context.

This guide should never be used as the sole prescription reference.

This book does not replace specialist formal education. This book is intended to clarify, inform, enlighten, and inspire its reader to seek more learning.

This guidebook is simply an introductory overview as a way for us all to have increased practical knowledgeable wisdom on the multiple options available to our clients – beyond the constraints and limitations of mainstream conventional medical obstetrics.

Note to Midwives

Personally, I completed my midwifery training in New Zealand, a country internationally renowned as arguably having the *best* maternity healthcare services in the world! I am a proud Kiwi midwife, knowing New Zealand is the only country on the planet that fulfils *all* the World Health Organization's recommendations for *best maternity services*, particularly via our continuity-of-care "Lead Maternity Carer" system. In past recent decades there has continued to be a steady improvement in our maternal and neonatal outcomes. In many ways we are doing an amazing job, especially for our medically complex patients. But particularly for our lower-risk clients, there are still many ways we could be doing things better.

Midwifery in particular (especially historically) has always recognized that complementary therapies such as herbalism can have significant influences on the normal progression of pregnancy and the spontaneous naturalness of childbirth, and give positive benefits during the postpartum, for both the woman and her baby. However, to quote the globally respected New Zealand College of Midwives, which sums things up succinctly: "Midwives incorporating these therapies into their practice should either have undertaken a recognised education programme or refer clients to appropriately qualified practitioners."

Midwives in general have *the* most unique role under the modern medicine banner. Yes, of course our knowledge is based on empirical science. But like no other role in medicine (close seconds: obstetricians and emergency medical staff), we are like the *Queens* of *intuitive healthcare*. When it's 5 a.m. at a homebirth and she's been pushing for 90 minutes, it is often our *gut instinct* we are observing the most (not just the fetal heart-rate and station of descent).

Special note: If you wish to be proudly known as a midwife who encourages women to embrace 'wholistic' modality wellness therapies, please do contact www.iimhco.com to register for our International Directory of IMHC-Friendly Midwives.

Note to Obstetricians

In New Zealand where I trained, midwives have full autonomy to manage all normal cares for the antepartum, intrapartum and postpartum. However, with increased-risk patients, we always liaise with our esteemed friends and appreciated colleagues (our wonderful obstetric doctors), who we will, on occasion, formally hand care over to temporarily for the management of their performing instrumental and surgical deliveries; and on rare occasions we will completely transfer care over to the obstetrics team for very high-risk, medically-complex pregnancies.

We value and appreciate our obstetric (and paediatric) colleagues tremendously; and in turn they value and admire us enormously as their midwifery colleagues and gurus of 'normal' (thus making us experts in recognizing when things are *not normal*).

It is a wonderful system – yet it too can certainly be improved, of course.

Just as there are decreasing numbers of old-school midwives who are a little too medicalized (e.g. just a little too quick with the third-stage ecbolic jab straight after a natural birth), we are also now seeing increasing numbers of new-school millennial obstetricians who are more holistically minded than ever before (and so a little less inclined to order the oxytocin drip just because the woman is only doing 5:20 contractions).

Note: If you wish to be proudly known as an obstetrician who encourages clients to embrace holistic modality wellness therapies as well as modern obstetric care-plans, please do contact www.iimhco.com to register for our International Directory of IMHC-Friendly Obstetricians.

Note to holistic Health Practitioners

We love you – especially when you're specializing in maternity and neonatal health!

As midwives and obstetricians, we need you too!

Women need you!

As the founding director of the IIMHCO Maternity Natural Health Symposiums and the IMHC Research e-Journal, I strongly ask you to please share, teach, train and educate us on your holistic perinatal therapeutic modalities. Please do know that many of us have immense respect for your contributions to maternal and neonatal wellness.

Note: If you are a holistic modality professional who specializes – or wishes to specialize – in maternity health and neonatal treatments, then please do contact www.iimhco.com to register for our International Directory of IMHC-Friendly Practitioners.

In summary ...

This introductory overview guidebook is akin to one centimetre of cervical dilatation, within the spectrum of formally giving birth to globally recognized and respected PIM best-practice guidelines.

This book is simply about kicking off the trend – around the world.

It is about breaking the ice into new uncharted waters – internationally.

It is about demanding into existence a new definition of "normal" – everywhere, collectively, "insynctively". So that eventually, holistic maternity health will become "mainstream" (normal, ordinary, conventional, and used by the local majority).

And one thing for absolute certainty is:

It WILL happen.

What we don't know yet is *when* it will happen or *where* – just like medicine globally, different countries will be at different paces.

In the end, it's only about changing perceptions. A belief is simply a thought we keep thinking.

Where half a century ago the "high, hot and a helleva lot" enemas were routine in obstetrics, now they're seen as barbaric. Thirty years ago, a woman choosing to keep her placenta was hippiedom Earth Mother extremist twaddle – yet now women routinely keep their placenta for a symbolic tree-planting burial, or encapsulation.

Times change. Societies evolve. We evolve.

So now today, we (author and reader) find ourselves jointly being pioneers into a time in the future, when we have fully realized our achievement of routine acceptance and embracement of the positive benefits of IMHCs/PIMs. And then you will tell tales to newly pregnant mothers-to-be, student midwives, and junior doctors, about how restricted and constricting past protocols were, and they will look at you wide-eyed as if to say options couldn't have really been so limited, surely not. To paraphrase my dear friend the renowned and incredible maternity anthropologist Dr Robbie Davis-Floyd, who summarizes medical evolution so succinctly:

> We have grown up with a technocratic model of medicine where the mind and body have been doctored separately, and with the body being treated like a malfunctioning machine often requiring aggressive intervention. *Technocratic* medicine has been a hierarchal organization striving to provide a standardization of care, and where diagnosis and treatment is provided from the outside in.

> In recent decades the public and practitioners have now demanded a more *humanistic* model of medicine, where the body as an organism is respected as having a mind-body connection, and where practitioners are expected to demonstrate caring compassion including obtaining informed consent decisions from their patients. Diagnosis and healing is provided from the outside in and from the inside out, with a focus on disease prevention. It has been science and technology counterbalanced with humanism and having an embryonic open-mindedness towards other modalities.

> But now, it is time for us to collectively advance things even further, to the next and ultimate level: the *holistic* model of medicine, where the objective is a oneness of mind-body-spirit, where the body is respected as an energy system, and where the goal is

treatment of the 'whole' person. Healing is primarily from the inside out, with individualized care, and with science and technology being at the service of the individual (who inherently has authority and responsibility over themselves). The overall focus is about creating long-term health and wellbeing, with multiple healing modalities embraced.

Today for expectant Millennial Gen-Ys (and soon our Alpha Gen-Z 'Zoomers'), along with their oftentimes consciously intentional healthy-lifestyle approaches, many want integrative medicine as mainstream to their birth journey – especially because labour is fundamentally both a science and a heart-based experience. Women, and commonly their partners too, are strongly desiring an integrational blending of modern obstetric medicine, with traditional naturopathic therapies, for they desire a healthcare approach that focuses holistically on the whole woman-baby dyad.

So just as the public are demanding more and more GPs be educated on integrative medicine, thus it is the obvious progression that our own specialty of maternity healthcare needs to do the same (become Integrated) – *and we are!*

> *The practice of complementary therapies by midwives, doulas, [obstetricians] and other care providers requires attention to the professional issues pertinent to integrating new – and somewhat alternative – strategies into mainstream maternity care.*
>
> *It is paramount that the introduction of one or more therapies is set in the context in which standard antenatal, intrapartum and postnatal care is delivered.*
>
> Denise Tiran, Complementary Therapies in Maternity Care

Overview Of Therapeutic Modalities

Overview of therapeutic modalities and their wellness supportive properties during the childbirth journey

Preamble

The more studies being done, then the more university research continues to confirm how incredibly popular naturopathic therapies are for expectant mothers all over the planet! Dozens of studies, one after another, are confirming that *most* mothers-to-be access complementary wellness of one kind or another during their maternity journey from a wide range of traditional and modern alternative modalities, rather than these women only relying on conventional allopathic obstetric biomedicine. That's just a fact. (Many of those specific research studies have been featured in the IMHC Research e-Journals – with back-copies available at www.iimhco.com.)

These many university researchers are commonly concluding that women use such wellness practices because they value the holistic natural approach, and they want greater participation in their own pregnancy care – even though empirical Western medicine has a scarce dearth of high-quality studies on natural medicinal treatment efficacies (pharmacokinetics, pharmacodynamics, etc.). Why? There are two significant barriers:

Firstly, lack of financial incentive: Big Pharma (who fund most drug research) cannot earn royalties on any substances found naturally in nature – they can only earn their patent income on synthetic molecules.

Secondly, lack of suitable empirical research techniques: homeopathy alone has around 50 different cough tinctures (that are all specific on the "whole picture" of the type of cough). So then how is it possible to run a double-blind randomized controlled trial on homeopathy with 50 different cough remedies? And what too of the many holistic healing modalities that specifically focus on the *triadic* human being (body-mind-spirit)?

All in all, it is incredibly challenging to create case-controlled quantitative studies which empiricism will respect and value (especially when historically one of its favourite accusations on anything different to itself is to label it "pseudo-science" even though the historic and anecdotal medical evidence is routinely enormous). Modern allopathic medicine has a Teflon-styled insulating layer of inherent arrogance it finds problematic to shed.

One thing that is quite clear, however, is that the two commonest complementary therapies midwives suggest to their clients is *acupuncture* and *homeopathy*. In fact, studies show around one-third of all midwives globally recommend homeopathy.

Today Western medicine is finally embracing Eastern acupuncture. So even though empirical science can't truly begin to scientifically prove *how* acupuncture works (lest we remind them its wellness works by restoring qi-energy meridian flows), they have finally accepted that it can provide miraculous therapeutic effects.

However, the vibrational tinctures of homeopathy can take empirical science way too far outside its current comfort-zone – even though quantum physics has proved humans are primarily *vibrational* beings that simply "appear" to be solid … when, in fact, at the end of the day, we are all simply atoms in a constant state of motion.

Just because you don't believe in something doesn't mean it isn't true.

Albert Einstein (1879–1955), theoretical physicist

Who or What are Naturopaths?

Naturopathy is an "umbrella term" as such.

Naturopaths are like the GPs (general practitioners) of HTMMs (holistic traditional and modern medicines).

They treat using various therapeutic modalities, dependent on what they've chosen to train in, but this nearly always includes medical herbalism of one or more type (e.g. Western, Chinese, Indian), and perhaps a manipulation therapy (e.g. acupuncture, osteopathy), and possibly employing alternative diagnostic tools (e.g. iridology, Neurolink®, live blood analysis); and typically naturopaths will have advanced knowledge or qualifications in nutrition.

Increasingly, naturopaths are also coming from a background of being a qualified doctor within the AMMA paradigm (allopathic modern medicine) who has grown disenchanted by their allopathic biomedical's inability to cure root causes of chronic dis-ease (and with Big Pharma's seeming obsession to only "cure" by suppressing symptoms rather than fixing the root cause). Let's face it, when you've been a modern medical doctor for a few years, it's hard not to become disillusioned that your best medical science actually doesn't have a clue on so much ... even how spontaneous childbirth labour commences (it only has theories). And it routinely prescribes thousands of drugs every day where the pharmacokinetics is officially "Action Unknown" ... heck, empirical science doesn't even know yet how to cure hiccups.

For increasing numbers of trail-blazing young MDs, they can find it repulsive to capitulate their worth becoming condensed down into becoming yet another "script-writing-machine" as they have witnessed many of their senior colleagues being. No, that is not for them! They want the boundaries between their work and their purpose to merge into one.

These free-thinking and forward-thinking, broad-minded and open-minded modern physicians can have a deep realization that truly progressive knowledge of medical healing is not originating from be-all and end-all synthetic pharmacology, but actually from the ageless and established; from the proven and corroborated; and from the ancient and anecdotal – not just the empirical double-blind randomized controlled trials.

WARNING

Do note the following therapies should not be used in life-threatening or high-risk situations in place of modern obstetric medical consultations and treatment management. However, many can be tremendously effective support during complex care.

Acupuncture/Acupressure/ Moxibustion

Special thanks to Janine Cuff of Mother-Well for her contribution to this introduction overview on acupuncture.

Acupuncture is an effective, highly developed and trusted holistic health system offering a safe and drug-free option in preconception, fertility and maternity healthcare. Within maternity wellness, acupuncture and acupressure are particularly associated with treating morning sickness or turning a breech baby, however it is capable of *much* more than that.

Acupuncture (and acupressure) has been used in China and other Eastern cultures for about 2500 years, to restore, promote and maintain good health and energy levels. Moxibustion is the traditional Chinese medicine that involves burning a moxa stick (mugwort) near a specific acupuncture point, such as encouraging a breech fetus to turn.

Acupuncturists seek not only to impart balance and restoration of health with the use of needles, moxibustion, heat, electro-stimulation, cupping, massage and acupressure, but also to empower through dietary education and lifestyle advice.

Treatments are preceded by a consultation process involving both medical science and traditional Chinese medicine perspectives. Not only do acupuncturists ask questions, they also look at the patient's skin, eyes, tongue, and how the body moves. They may palpate (examine by touch) relevant local and distal areas of the body for temperature, tension, swellings or abnormalities, plus they will gather further information from the pulse.

Acupuncture offers a wide range of healing and support along the entire maternity journey. The regular contact (and sometimes just the chance to lie down, relax, and vent in the middle of our busy modern life) can offer reassurance, physical attention, and much needed mental and emotional support. Such reduction in tension and stress leads to improved comfort, mental function and vitality … a great base for any healing process.

Preconception and fertility

During preconception and fertility care the focus of the acupuncturist working with couples is to support and balance the reproductive and digestive systems and regulate sympathetic stress responses. Acupuncturists educate their clients in the understanding of the menstrual cycle and sperm health; establish the fertile window; and optimize the reproductive system through nutrition and lifestyle advice.

If fertility issues are evident, acupuncturists work closely to regulate and restore hormone balance, offering treatments for multiple disorders, including PCOS, endometriosis, dysmenorrhea, amenorrhea, pre-menstrual symptoms, irregularity, and multiple miscarriages. Additionally, they offer IVF treatment support.

Pregnancy

During pregnancy, acupuncturists commonly would be seen weekly in the beginning four to eight weeks depending on wellbeing, then again in the final four weeks of pregnancy in the lead-up to labour; plus in-between usually monthly visits, or as required, depending on how the pregnancy and comfort levels are progressing.

Throughout the first trimester, acupuncturists mainly focus on the digestive system, nutrient and blood flow to the uterus, stress relief and general wellbeing. Treatments often focus on these issues: miscarriage support, morning sickness, insomnia, stress, headaches, and tiredness.

During the second and into the third trimester, pregnancy issues arising commonly treated with acupuncture include: restless legs, muscle cramps, back pain, heartburn reflux, swellings, carpal tunnel syndrome, pelvic/pubic pain, sinus troubles, coughs/colds, elevated blood pressure, and reduced fetal growth (small for dates). Treatments are often focused on the reduction of tension, inflammation and pain in the tissues and mucous membranes; plus increasing local blood flow, and nervous system support.

Very specific to acupuncture and moxibustion is the treatment of fetal malposition (e.g. posterior) and malpresentation (e.g. breech). Optimal timing for treatments is 34 weeks but can be used as late as 39- weeks. Alongside acupuncture, treatment with moxibustion is commonly taught in clinics to be used by the woman in her home over a period of 10 days.

Labour preparation

From week 36, acupuncture preparations for labour begin, along with continuation of holistic support as required. Often at this stage commonly presenting symptoms include swelling lower limbs, lower back pain, hip pain, leg cramps, and anxiety. Alongside treatments, acupressure points are explained, taught, marked and demonstrated for use at home, both in the preparation for childbirth, and for use by the woman's support partner during labour.

Acupressure points are often found to be extremely effective in pain management and in hastening the onset and progression of establishing strong, productive, active labour. They can also be very useful to aid a natural birth and onset of contractions, in situations where labour induction is medically indicated, such as AMA (advanced maternal age), GDM (gestational diabetes mellitus), PE (pre-eclampsia), overdue post-dates (42+ weeks), or other pregnancy complications.

Often at these stressful times, after acupuncture women comment about how empowered they feel, especially when including home treatments using acupressure. This gain in confidence creates a feeling of relaxation that in turn results in a sense of wellbeing.

Postpartum support

The first five to six weeks of mothering a newborn can often be a difficult (virtually impossible) time for new mothers to visit an acupuncturist's clinic, especially if they have had to undergo a caesarean section. Where possible some acupuncturists will be happy to arrange a home visit.

Common issues supported by acupuncture at this time, and over the following weeks, include tiredness, breastfeeding support, uterine prolapse, urinary disorders, haemorrhoids, poor memory, night sweats, scar healing, insomnia, stress, anxiety, and depression.

Also, it is often a good time to teach the parents newborn acupressure and massage techniques to help their baby with digestive discomfort, cough, colic, reflux, sleep, wind, crying and restlessness.

What acupuncture, acupressure and moxibustion can treat (but not limited to):

- Nausea and vomiting (pregnancy morning sickness and during labour)
- High/low blood pressure
- Diabetes
- Tiredness and fatigue
- Constipation, diarrhoea, irritable bowel
- Tender breasts
- Migraine and other headaches
- Backache, sciatica
- Pelvic girdle pain (e.g. symphysis pubis dysfunction)
- Carpel tunnel
- Varicose veins (e.g. legs, vulva)
- Haemorrhoids
- Insomnia
- Mental health issues (e.g. anxiety)
- Heartburn, acid reflux, indigestion
- Low-lying placenta
- Oedema (swelling)
- Birth preparation (e.g. cervical ripening)
- Fetal malposition and malpresentation (i.e. moxibustion to turn a breech baby)
- Natural labour induction

- Pain relief during labour
- Acceleration of contractions (labour augmentation)
- Retained placenta
- General wellness recovery from childbirth
- Lactation and breast engorgement
- Prevention and treatment of postnatal depression

Ayurveda Medicine (Indian Herbalism)

Ayurvedic healthcare is a system of medicinal preparations and surgical procedures that has its historical roots in Vedic (Hindu) India. It is a medicinal system that has evolved over more than two thousand years, and potentially much earlier (scholarly opinion varies as it being 4000 to 6000 years old). Like all ancient healing, therapies are dominantly based on herbal and mineral substances.

Later in history, some of the non-Vedic systems on the Indian subcontinent, such as Buddhism and Jainism, also developed medical practices based on classical Ayurveda texts.

Today Ayurveda is still immensely respected in India, Nepal and Sri Lanka, plus it has been well and truly globalized into the modern Western world, with practices commonly integrated into general wellness applications.

Ayurveda treatises are based on three elemental dosha ("doṣa") forces called *vāta*, *pitta* and *kapha*; then within these three doshas are five sub-categories to each. Ayurvedic medicine teaches that equality (equilibrium) of the doṣas (termed *sāmyatva*) results in homeostatic (balanced) health – and that inequality imbalance (termed *viṣamatva*) results in dis-ease.

Under Ayurveda, well-recommended pregnancy healthcare includes oil full-body self-massage and foot massage, walking, swimming, preggy-yoga, meditation, rest, pure water, controlled breath, sunshine, loving respectful relationships, positive joyful thoughts, and of course vital foodstuffs – all in an effort to maintain and restore the *Apana Vāta* balance (the downward-moving flow of energy in the body, including urination and elimination).

The three ancient Ayurvedic pregnancy self-care guidelines

EAT FRESH COOKED FOODS: e.g. avoiding processed or leftover reheated food – and when pregnant, cooked food is better for digestion than raw food. Such "pure" foods that provide *prana* (cosmic life-force) include organic dairy, nuts, wholegrains, beans, fruit and fresh cooked vegetables.

INCLUDE HEALTHY DIETARY FATS AND OILS: e.g. whole milk, coconut oil, olive oil, nuts, seeds, avocado, and cooking with ghee (clarified butter). Also, because so many herbs are fat-soluble, consuming them with healthy fats improves delivery of cellular nutrition. A particularly healthy evening drink during pregnancy is a glass of warm milk with a teaspoon of ghee and half a teaspoon each of turmeric and cardamom powders, to improve digestion, calm nerves, and to aid sleep.

OIL MASSAGE: Daily self-massage to nourish your mind and love your body (as well as the baby's spirit).

Daily pregnancy nutrition

From an iron tonic to herbal medicines, Ayurveda provides a great alternative for pregnant women in place of routine over-the-counter nutritional supplements. Ayurveda also assists to modulate the immune system, including antimicrobial actions.

Ayurvedic herbs commonly used in pregnancy

NETTLE LEAVES: High in vitamins A, C, K, calcium, potassium and iron, nettle leaves ease leg-cramp muscle-spasms, reduce haemorrhoids, aid the kidneys, decrease labour and postpartum contraction pain, prevent postpartum haemorrhage, and increase breastmilk richness.

RED RASPBERRY LEAVES: Containing the alkaloid *fragrine*, red raspberry leaves used in the third trimester assist to tone the uterine muscles to help reduce pre-term labour, labour contraction pain, and postpartum haemorrhage; plus can increase breastmilk production.

DANDELION LEAVES: Rich in calcium and folic acid, dandelion leaves promote general wellbeing, improve appetite, reduce skin complaints, heal and nourish the liver, help kidney function, provide a good source of calcium and potassium, and can relieve mild oedema. For pre-eclampsia, it is recommended to consume about 3–4 ounces (approximately 100g) a day of fresh or cooked dandelion leaves.

OATS AND OATSTRAW: Both oats and oatstraw are rich in calcium and magnesium, and can be consumed to promote a strong endocrine and nervous systems, helping to relieve irritated skin, inflammation, spasms, restlessness and anxiety. Oatstraw is also excellent to rejuvenate women during the postpartum from feeling quite so tired and weak.

ASHWAGANDHA: This is a great herb for women feeling weak during their pregnancy, and it is also said to help stabilize the fetus.

SHATAVARI: A nutritious herb great for the reproductive system, and as a rejuvenating nerve tonic.

NOTE: Sadly, it has been discovered that around 20 per cent of Ayurvedic medicines sold online have been found to contain toxic levels of heavy metals. Thus, seeing a classically qualified Ayurvedic doctor's practice is strongly preferable over self-diagnosing with online remedies.

Bach's Flower Essences (Including Rescue Remedy)

Bach flower remedies are 38 flower essences discovered and categorized by London physician Dr Edward Bach using a similar (though different) vibrational principle to homeopathy. The remedies extract the flower essences into spring water, then brandy is added as a preservative, and the mixture diluted for medicinal use.

This type of remedy is very safe, because empirically it does not contain any chemicals, except a very small amount of alcohol. (They are closer to "vibrational" tinctures than herbal remedies.)

Bach's flower remedies treat the body on an emotional level, to alleviate unhappy feelings and unblock the body's natural restorative abilities. The essences can be incredibly effective, and are especially wonderful for assisting with anxiety, shock, trauma (including the birth support people too); and in fact anyone feeling anxious or under pressure. They will promote calm; reduce fretful/irritable feelings; and can be beautifully used in conjunction with other remedies (such as homeopathy).

During the maternity journey, Bach's flower essences can be especially helpful with general pregnancy relaxation including relief of stress and anxiety, plus general recovery from childbirth labour, and as part of the prevention/ treatment of postnatal depression.

Rescue Remedy

Perhaps the most famous of Bach's combination preparations "Rescue Remedy" is an essential for the household first-aid kit. It encourages immediate calm and emotional stabilizing, and is good for recovery from frights, shocks, arguments, anxiety, irritability, nightmares, and overtired sleeplessness.

NOTE: It is an especially excellent strategy for women to include a few drops of Rescue Remedy in their water bottle throughout labour and birth.

Individual BACH® Remedies

- Agrimony – reduces inner turmoil to communicate openly
- Aspen – reduces apprehension to feel secure
- Beech – reduces intolerance to accept imperfections
- Centaury – increases assertiveness to be able to say 'No'
- Cerato – reduces self-doubt to trust your own intuition
- Cherry Plum – encourages clarity during chaos to be in control
- Chestnut Bud – assists to learn from mistakes to move forward
- Chicory – helps you take a step back, and love unconditionally
- Clematis – encourages concentration to stay focused
- Crab Apple – encourages embracing yourself to accept imperfections
- Elm – reduces feelings of being overwhelmed, to maintain assured perspective
- Gentian – helps coping with challenging difficulties by

putting setbacks into perspective

- Gorse – helps to find the positive sunshine despite dark problems to have hope
- Heather – encourages positive communication to empathize and listen
- Holly – encourages generous goodwill towards others without judgment
- Honeysuckle – helps to embrace the now by leaving regret in the past
- Hornbeam – helps to cope with facing the day's challenges ahead, to procrastinate less
- Impatiens – reduces impatience to find ease with less haste
- Larch – reduces nerves by boosting inner confidence
- Mimulus – reduces fears to encourage positive potential
- Mustard – brings joy back into a gloomy day
- Oak – recharges exhaustion to restore endurance
- Olive – revitalizes and restores mental energy
- Pine – encourages self-respect by reducing self-blame
- Red Chestnut – reduces anxiety to give peace of mind
- Rock Rose – reduces helpless panic to give calm courage
- Rock Water – inhibits inflexibility to have an open attitude
- Scleranthus – encourages certainty by reducing indecisiveness
- Star of Bethlehem – soothes sorrow giving inner strength
- Sweet Chestnut – reduces hopeless despair to regain peace of mind
- Vervain – gives serenity, wisdom and tolerance for relaxed calm
- Vine – motivates determination, without domination
- Walnut – assists handling life changes by improving

adaptability
- Water Violet – allows you to cultivate connections with others
- White Chestnut – calms the mind to give tranquil peace
- Wild Oat – helps gives inner clarity to decide on the right path
- Wild Rose – increases enthusiasm to take initiative and make life changes
- Willow – combats victim resentment to forgive and forget

Bowen Therapy

Special thanks to Australian trainer and practitioner Katrina Ridley for her contribution to this introduction overview on Bowen Therapy.

The relaxing, subtle and painless *Bowen Therapy* was developed by Thomas Bowen in Geelong, Victoria, Australia in the 1950s. Bowen shared his therapy to a handful of people, one of which was Oswald Rentsch. In 1986 Mr Rentsch decided he would teach others what has become known as Bowen Therapy. As a result of these beginnings Bowen Therapy is now found worldwide. Bowen Therapy is a gentle, effective, non-invasive body therapy.

The effectiveness of Bowen Therapy lends itself to promoting wellbeing and relief from discomfort for the infant, the frail and aged, and everyone in between. The evidence for the efficacy of Bowen Therapy is anecdotal and there is a large amount of it.

It needs to be noted that every person and therefore every person's physical body responds differently to any intervention, and how people respond to Bowen is no different. Bowen Therapy has and continues to help people achieve improved health and wellbeing at multiple levels.

What Bowen Therapy can treat (but not limited to):

PRE-CONCEPTION HEALTH: Bowen techniques can improve fertility through helping the body to find balance. (It can also be a good idea to treat the partner too. Plus, Bowen is also helpful for IVF success.)

PREGNANCY HEALTH: Bowen techniques are able to help ensure wellbeing, by assisting the body to find and maintain wellness, including: gestational diabetes, cholestasis, recurrent vaginosis; breast mammogenesis pain; reducing recurrent miscarriages; colds, flus, hay fever, rhinitis (assists congestion drainage); constipation and diarrhoea; balancing intense emotions; improving exhaustion fatigue energy levels; relief of indigestion heartburn; effective to assist carpal tunnel syndrome, leg cramps, sciatica, SPD; and improving insomnia, palpitations and depression by helping the body to relax and move from sympathetic to parasympathetic dominated.

LABOUR AND BIRTH CARE: Bowen has been used all over the world during labour and birth because their techniques can be helpful to ease both the first and second stages by helping the woman to feel relaxed and calm, including improvements to her levels of hydration, exhaustion, fear and shock. Plus, the 'Coccyx Procedure' can be helpful in the third stage.

MATERNAL POSTPARTUM: Potentially helpful for many issues, particularly assisting to reduce bonding/blues depression/anxiety, and insomnia. Plus, Bowen has a good perineal procedure that is helpful to those women who experience post-episiotomy referred pain.

NEONATAL: Bowen techniques often have great results for colic, reflux, wind and constipation; plus, recovery from long labours and traumatic deliveries, especially calming and relaxing the newborn.

Chiropractic

There is general lack of understanding of the differences between *chiropractic* and *osteopathy*, because both work on the musculoskeletal system (bones, joints, ligaments, tendons) and both work on the neurological system (that influences other body systems). Their philosophies are similar, but as a general summary of the unique difference: osteopathy considers the whole body treating a wide range of conditions, whereas chiropractic focuses mainly on spinal realignment and the neurological system to prevent and treat organ-function compromise. Chiropractic treatments tend to be short but frequent, and osteopathy treatments tend to be longer and more spaced out.

Modern lifestyles can make spinal communication systems dysfunctional due to postural stresses, altered spinal curves, misalignment, joint restrictions, and imbalances in the surrounding muscles ligaments and other tissues. However, from newborns to the elderly patients, the chiropractic philosophy is simple: *If the nervous system is working properly, then the whole body can heal quicker and perform better.*

Chiropractic is about the detection and correction of daily stresses and strains on the spine and its soft tissue (termed *vertebral subluxations*) to reduce their consequential blockages to the nervous system (which is encased by the spine, and which controls the body's functions), so that messages can reach organs more effectively to enhance function and overall health. Chiropractic care can benefit all aspects of the body's ability to be healthy by optimizing brain-body communication through the nervous system.

The purpose of chiropractic examination is to assess the spine and nervous system functioning and locate any areas of subluxations, and diagnosis can include observation (e.g. posture, gait, range of motion); palpation (touching the muscle tension and feeling joint mobility); routine orthopaedic and neurological tests; blood-tests and urinalysis; and oftentimes imaging (e.g. spinal X-ray, MRI scans).

Popular for maternity back pain and to encourage breech babies to turn, chiropractic recognizes that altered spinal structure and neurological function during pregnancy can have profound effects in expectant women resulting in their experiencing more discomfort during their pregnancy. Research evidence routinely shows chiropractic can reduce the woman's need for pharmaceuticals in the crucial time leading up to birth, including needing less assisted labours (fewer epidurals = fewer oxytocin drips), thus assisting to make giving birth an easier and safer experience for both the mother and baby.

Conditions chiropractic can assist with during the maternity journey (but not limited to):

- Overall maintaining of a healthy pregnancy
- Controlling symptoms of nausea and vomiting during pregnancy and labour
- Relieving back, neck and joint pain, including sciatica and pelvic girdle pain
- Heartburn, acid reflux, indigestion
- Constipation, diarrhoea, irritable bowel
- Haemorrhoids
- Varicosities (legs, vulva)

- Oedema
- Carpel tunnel
- Birth preparation reducing length of labour and birth, and consequently preventing a potential emergency C-section
- Fetal malposition and malpresentation (Webster's technique for breech babies)
- General recovery from childbirth

Essential Oils/Aromatherapy

Special thanks to journalist, Women's Holistic Wellness Practitioner, and Holistic Beauty Editor Shannon Dunn for her contribution to this introduction overview on essential oils.

Essential oils are natural aromatic compounds found in the seeds, bark, stems, roots, flowers and other parts of plants – with potential exquisite and powerful fragrances. Essential oils can lift a mood, calm the senses, and elicit powerful emotional responses – but they can also have profound health benefits therapeutically and medicinally, including many oils being naturally antimicrobial and/or cleansing.

Certified pure essential oils are powerfully concentrated, and their wellbeing vitality is usually administered by one of two methods during pregnancy:

- Diffused aromatically (i.e. aromatherapy)
- Applied topically (diluting the essential oil with a carrier oil, such as fractionated coconut oil).

Important points to note

Always appropriately dilute essential oils before use with a pure carrier oil. A favourite carrier oil is fractionated coconut oil because it has the fats removed and so is a thinner oil, thereby allowing better absorption of the essential oils through the skin and into the bloodstream. Another popular carrier oil is cold-pressed sweet almond.

Essential oils should never be used in the eyes or ear canal.

If skin irritation occurs, dilute by applying a vegetable oil to the area (water does not dilute oil).

Get what you pay for

It is critical to appreciate that "essential oils" can vary drastically in their quality (and thus their effectiveness).

For the highest quality, both meticulous harvesting and exacting extraction methods are required to create the purest therapeutic or tested grade essential oils, which generally involves low-heat steam distillation to create the superior quality (the oils are then also subjected to rigorous mass spectrometry and gas chromatography testing to ensure composition).

"You get what you pay for" rings extremely true for essential oils, and for the safest and most beneficial oils you are best to seek out reputable brands able to state their oils are "100% Pure Tested Grade". We recommend opting for a manufacturer such as dōTERRA® who produce pure, beyond organic, essential oils, with single-source origins and rigorous batch-testing and certifications to back them up.

The CPTG (Certified Pure Tested Grade) quality protocol includes the following regimes: organoleptic testing; microbial testing; gas chromatography; mass spectrometry; FTIR (Fourier Transform Infrared spectroscopy); chirality testing; Isotopic analysis; and heavy metal testing.

Essential oils during pregnancy

Pregnancy can represent an ideal opportunity for women to

take advantage of the safe benefits of using essential oils, plus it can enable them to have some control over the numerous physiological and emotional changes causing secondary issues such as morning sickness. It is empowering to have timely and effective solutions.

There are many essential oils that are wonderfully supportive during pregnancy, however, women should also always listen to their own body and intuition throughout each trimester. Using a diffuser (i.e. aromatherapy) is a wonderful way to receive essential oil benefits in a very gentle manner.

Essential oils are highly concentrated substances, so during pregnancy, *less is more* because there can be heightened sensitivity when women are pregnant. Thus, the golden rule: *Always dilute essential oils before use and only use oils you know with certainty are 100 per cent pure.*

Oils to avoid during pregnancy

Fennel, marjoram, tarragon, caraway, cinnamon, thuja, mugwort, birch, wintergreen, basil, camphor, hyssop, aniseed, sage, tansy, wormwood, parsley seed or leaf, pennyroyal, nutmeg, rosemary, jasmine, sage, tea tree, peppermint, eucalyptus and juniper berry.

Women should always listen to their intuition. If any oil does not feel right for her, she should err on the side of caution.

Special note: CLARY SAGE OIL

It is best to regard Clary Sage as "Mother Nature's oxytocin", making in contraindicated in these situations:

- *Prior to 37–38 weeks' gestation*
- *Well-established labour contractions*
- *Excessive lochia discharge*
- *RPOC (retained products of conception i.e. retained placenta)*
- *Woman receiving uterine stimulant (e.g. Syntocinon drip)*
- *Birth attendants/staff in the room who are pregnant*

Favourite blends for infant massage

- Melaleuca essential oil, combined with a quality massage blend (such as dōTERRA® "AromaTouch", which combines cypress, peppermint, marjoram, basil, grapefruit and lavender).
- Author personal favourite for inexpensive infant massage oil: few drops of lavender pure essential oil in a bottle of cold-pressed almond oil.

Conditions aromatherapy can assist with during the maternity journey (but not limited to):

- Morning sickness, nausea and indigestion heartburn
- Back discomfort, including lower back, sciatica, legs and feet
- Better sleep (insomnia)
- Skin changes and oedema
- Pregnancy calming and uplifting emotional support
- Tiredness, fatigue
- Constipation, diarrhoea, irritable bowel
- Birth preparation (e.g. cervical ripening)

- During childbirth, reducing tense stress, increasing positivity, easing lower back discomfort, balancing emotions, dispelling anxiety, soothing the mind, relaxing the body through back/shoulder massage – and generally helpful to mental health issues.
- Natural labour induction and accelerations of contractions
- Pain relief during labour
- General recovery from childbirth
- Wound healing and infection
- Breast engorgement
- Prevention/treatment of postnatal depression

Homeopathy

Homeopathy with good dietary advice, exercise and optimal positioning of baby attributed to my 90% normal uncomplicated birth rates. I stopped homeopathy for a while focusing upon dietary advice and exercise, but my assisted birth statistics increased. When I recommenced the use of homeopathy, the need for assisted birth reduced.

Irene Chain Kalinowski, British-NZ midwife/author and senior maternity/homeopathy educator

Homeopathic remedies harness the potent therapeutic properties of plants, animals and minerals to stimulate the body to heal itself into health. The medicines are prepared to exacting pharmacopeia standards and are prescribed very differently from mainstream medicine, and are an especially gentle way to treat every level: mental, emotional, physical, spiritual.

Homeopathy was developed as a system of medicine by respected German physician, scholar, scientist and teacher Dr Samuel Hahnemann (1755-1843) in the nineteenth century, based on the "like cures like" principle, combined with treating dis-ease by holistic diagnosis (the "whole person"), and with the fundamental principle of administrating the smallest doses of medicine possible. The word *homeopathy* simple brings together the two Greek words *homeo* (meaning similar/like) and *pathos* (meaning disease/suffering). (Interestingly, modern vaccine inoculations also work on the *like cures like* science to trigger the body creating immunity.)

Hahnemann's research was never an entirely brand-new

concept. More than 2000 years earlier, Hippocrates (the father of modern medicine) also subscribed to the "like cures like" philosophy of a medicine matching the illness symptoms (for example, using onion to treat hay-fever symptoms of runny, itchy nose and eyes). Hahnemann resurrected these principles and devoted his life to developing, researching and testing substances to make the like-for-like smallest-dose-possible medicines, now known as *homeopathic tinctures.*

Unappreciated by many Western pharmacologists, homeopathy is actually very well respected internationally, especially in UK/Europe and the Indian subcontinent. History hasn't forgotten that 1830 saw an 80 per cent recovery of homeopathic patients during the cholera epidemic. Or that by 1850, homeopathy was being used to successfully treat yellow fever, scarlet fever and typhoid fever. By 1900 America alone had 22 homeopathic medical schools, over 100 homeopathic hospitals, around 1000 homeopathic pharmacies, and about 15,000 homeopathic practitioners. Following the lead of midwives, obstetric doctors at the time and their "accoucheurs" (obstetric assistants) were also commonly using homeopathy as part of their practice.

One hundred years ago in the 1920s, modern Western allopathic medicine began to get a real foothold, and pharmaceuticals began the systematic condemnation of homeopathy. Today, any Westerners who know practically nothing about homeopathy yet still strongly regard it as hocus-pocus pseudoscience quackery, demonstrate first-hand just how powerful the propaganda spin machine remains, even a century on.

Homeopathy is well documented to assist with many general

medical issues, including chronic and infectious diseases, multiple first-aid situations, all varieties of emotional stress, plus learning and behavioural disorders including addiction.

In reality, homeopathy remains mainstream in many countries around the world. The British royal family are firm users of homeopathy, including the UK still having homeopathic hospitals attached to the NHS, and homeopathy remains Europe's most popular alternative medicine to allopathic Western medicine, with nearly 30 per cent of European citizens using homeopathy as their go-to OTC (over-the-counter) healthcare. In fact, almost one-third of French physicians prescribe homeopathy as part of their practice, and nearly 100 per cent of all German pharmacies stock homeopathy.

Homeopathy remains a non-toxic and inexpensive "energy" vibrational medicine, a cousin, you could say, to acupuncture, Chinese and Ayurveda medicines (and in fact most indigenous medical systems), which all practise triadic wellness of the interconnection between mind and body health.

Homeopathic remedies are vibrational dilutions that start out as a mother-tincture – then the higher the dilution, the more pure the energy (a concept empirical pharmaceutical medicine finds impossible to grasp). Another unique difference with homeopathic remedies is that they should only be taken for symptomatic conditions – they are not designed to be taken prophylactically (i.e. as a preventative).

Today homeopathy provides effective first-line treatment for millions globally. And like midwifery, its practice is both "an art and a science" – and I must recommend that all birth practitioners become familiar with their local homeopathic dispensing pharmacy.

Overview guidelines

- The commonest potencies are 30C and 200C ... think of 30C for minor/chronic conditions, and 200C for acute care.
- With over 50 different remedies for just a cough, the "right remedy" is discerned by considering the "holistic" (whole picture) of that person. The right remedy cures (reduces symptoms) with no nasty side effects. When the wrong remedy is given, there are no side effects, and no cure – it has no effect ... and this is again a very difficult concept for modern pharmacology to understand where for pharmacists *every* medication (mostly synthetic molecules) produce side effects (that is their purpose: to be prescribed for their desired predicted side effect, with the hope of not causing too many undesired predictable adverse reactions.)
- Classical homeopaths match symptom-picture of the person with symptom-personality of the remedy. However, today much of the work is already done for us, e.g. Arnica for bruising. Why Arnica? Many regular users have little idea, but simply know it works.
- Homeopathy works on an "administer as little as needed until change is effected" basis. Subsequent constant symptom changes are an excellent sign too, which can sometimes require a change in remedy as the unwellness progresses through its various stages of healing (often compared to "peeling layers off an onion" to get to the root cause of outward symptoms). Even an initial momentary increase in a symptom is often a

positive sign that can occur, then rapidly the patient begins to feel better.

- *Chronic/non-acute dose:* typically, 2 drops 3–4 times a day orally, or 4–6 drops in cup of warm water sipped throughout the day, repeated as necessary until improvement.
- *Acute dose:* every 5–15 minutes.
- Drops/sprays (in an alcohol base) or pilules (tiny sugar tablets) are all administered sublingually (under the tongue) to be absorbed systemically by the mucosal tissue into the bloodstream (for better efficacy than swallowing the dose into the digestive system).

Conditions homeopathy can assist with during the maternity journey (but not limited to):

- History of miscarriages
- General pregnancy relaxation and relief of stress/anxiety
- Mental health issues (e.g. anxiety and depressive disorders)
- Pregnancy headaches
- Oedema (fluid imbalance)
- Nausea and vomiting (morning sickness and during labour)
- Heartburn (including acid reflux, indigestion)
- Hay fever, asthma and eczema (and other skin disorders)
- Backache, sciatica
- Pelvic, muscle and ligament discomforts including separated symphysis
- Haemorrhoids
- Varicosities (legs and vulva)
- Cholestasis (should never replace obstetric

management)
- Coughs/colds/earaches/influenza (boosts lowered immune system)
- Carpel tunnel syndrome
- Exhaustion, tiredness, fatigue
- Insomnia and sleeplessness
- Recurrent UTIs (and other infections)
- Birth preparation (cervical ripening, strengthening uterine muscles, toning uterine shape, improving fetal position and descent, removing maternal fears and anxieties)
- Physiological process of labour and birth (natural induction of labour and acceleration of contractions)
- Reducing childbirth complications (e.g. encouraging a breech baby to turn, and as pain-relief during labour)
- Retained placenta
- Wound healing
- Improving general postpartum recovery from birth
- Lactation and breast engorgement
- Postnatal depression
- Infants: neonatal transition from intrauterine to extrauterine life, skin disorders, ear infections, colic, reflux, discontent disposition (excessive crying) and poor weight-gain – plus much more.

Homeopathy does not tout itself as the cure-all to severe disease. It does, however, proudly know itself to perhaps be the ultimate definition of a complementary medicine which can be used beautifully in conjunction with any and all other naturopathic and allopathic treatments.

A useful analogy can be to regard homeopathy as a "support system". Now oftentimes, that "support", when used as the first cab off the rank, can result in no further supportive treatments being required. Homeopathy has never represented itself as always being the *only* form of medicine required.

Just as Band-Aids can oftentimes be the only treatment needed to heal a wound, and are also well known to speed the body's natural healing, so too homeopathy can oftentimes be the only treatment needed, with its innate ability to enhance the body's natural healing capabilities.

Insistently arguing that homeopathy should never be solely relied upon for the treatment of all disease is as an intelligent a statement as decreeing Band-Aids should never be solely relied upon for the treatment of all wounds. Band-Aids have never stated they are the only wound-care treatment necessary – just as homeopathy has never stated it is the only disease-care treatment necessary.

Essential Tinctures For Birth Practitioners

These are the eight remedies all Birth Practitioners should know the scope of use of, for the antepartum, intrapartum and postpartum:

- Gelsemium
- Bellis
- Pulsatilla
- Sepia
- Arnica
- Caulophyllum
- Kali Carb
- Cimicifuga
- OTHER USEFUL REMEDIES TO CARRY: Aconite, Arsenicum, Hypercal, Kali phos, Pyrogen and

Staphysagria

NOTE: Strong aromas will act as an antidote making the homeopathic tinctures inactive (i.e. ineffectual), such as essential oils, mint, spiced foods, toothpaste, chewing gum, eucalyptus decongestants, cough lozenges and coffee.

Hypnotherapy

Hypnotherapy is a natural yet altered state of consciousness, in which the critical part of the mind is quietened and access is given to the most powerful part of the subconscious mind. During this altered state our brain is extremely active, which has been documented and measured through PET, MRI and detailed EEG scans. Generally, the hypnotherapist uses deep relaxation and focused concentration to assist people into the hypnotic state. Hypnotherapy is a safe and powerful tool for enhancing focus and overcoming psychosomatic issues, unwanted habits, phobias, feelings of uneasiness and self-esteem issues.

Ideal general uses include enhancing study/learning, concentration and sports performance; anaesthesia/pain-relief management (chronic, surgical or dental pain-relief); breaking unwanted dysfunctional habits such as smoking, overeating and nail-biting; and modifying emotional behaviour, such as anxiety. Hypnotherapists will also sometimes combine NLP (neuro-linguistic programming) as one of their tools.

Conditions hypnotherapy can assist with during the maternity journey (but not limited to):

- General pregnancy relaxation (relief of stress/anxiety)
- Mental health Issues (anxiety, depression)
- Tiredness, fatigue
- Birth preparation (mental empowerment)
- Pain relief during labour (deep-relaxation self-hypnosis

termed *hypnobirthing*, or what I call "meditative labour"
– refer Part Three, Intrapartrum (Labour and Birth)
· General recovery from childbirth
· Preventing/treatment of postnatal depression
· Hypnotherapy may also be able to assist with nausea,
  vomiting; constipation, diarrhoea, irritable bowel; fetal
  malposition/malpresentation; and natural labour
  induction.

Massage

Pregnancy massage during the antenatal period is nothing new, and history is full of traditional cultures all over the planet who have practised maternity massage, from Jamaica to Japan, and from Mexico to Malaysia. Massage during the antenatal period is similar to non-pregnant massage in that it soothes sore and achy muscles – the main difference is that the masseuse should be trained in the simple modifications (mainly positional) needed to ensure the safety and comfort of both the mother and the unborn baby.

Women in childbirth labour have received massage for hundreds of thousands of years, and is a practice likely as old as humankind! There are primarily two reasons massage during labour can feel so good:

- Firstly, in physiology the Gate Theory is the point that generally one dominant message of sensation travels up the spine to the brain – which is why, when we stub our toe, our immediate instinct is to rub our toe (so that the rubbing sensation overrides the pain sensation). The principle is exactly the same with massage during labour (or using a TENS machine during contractions): the massage (or transcutaneous electrical nerve stimulation) becomes the dominant message to the brain, effectively "drowning out" the sharpness of the contraction pain. *Women often during labour want hours and hours of gentle massage across their lower back and sacrum, which acts as an effective distraction.*
- Secondly, deep massage that is borderline painful acts as something termed a DNIC (diffuse noxious inhibitory

control) method of pain relief of "pain inhibits pain". The principle is that this very intense massage stimulates the brain to release pain-relieving endorphins, which creates the side effect of perceiving contractions to be less intense. Women often during labour will insist their birth support person massages them "Harder, harder!", with men particularly often taken aback by just how firm their partner is demanding the massage to be, especially, I have witnessed, with hip-compression squeezes.

- And thirdly, logically, of course, massage must decrease stress cortisol, thus increasing serotonin and dopamine.

Multiple research studies have concluded massage during labour produces lower pain scores typically by a couple of points (particularly during the transition phase); plus, less anxiety; an increased sense of control; and generally higher rates of overall birth experience satisfaction.

In general terms, from personally witnessing hundreds and hundreds of natural labours and normal births, I have noticed the following cascade as the general time lapse of what I'll term:

Labour's stages of massage

- Early–mid latent labour (mild–moderate 30–45 second contractions every 5–10 minutes): No massage is best (intentionally reserving it as a pain reliever for later).
- Late latent labour (stronger contractions every 4–5 minutes): Birth support person commences using "effleurage" (skimming light-touch strokes) during contractions only (not in-between).

- Established active labour (3–4 strong contractions every 10 minutes, all 60–90 seconds long): Birth support person uses sacral lower-back counter-pressure, increasing in intensity as dilatation increases, fully directed by the woman instructing her needs and desires.
- Transitional advanced labour (4–5 very strong and long contractions every 10 minutes, and 8–9 cm dilatated): Birth support person using very strong hip squeezes ("rounding" the oval-shape pelvic outlet providing anatomical relief, and such sensation providing DNIC pain-inhibiting-pain).
- Second stage (fully dilatated and pushing): No massage – it can seem to all become too distracting for the woman.

NB: The above is a generalization – every unmedicated labour is unique, so best guided by the woman herself. She will know her needs at the time.

Conditions massage can assist with during the maternity journey (but not limited to):

- General pregnancy relaxation (reduces stress)
- Relieves joint pain and sore muscles
- Relieves headaches
- Mental health issues (anxiety, depression)
- Tiredness, fatigue
- Insomnia (improves sleep)
- Constipation, diarrhoea, irritable bowel
- Heartburn
- Haemorrhoids
- Reduces oedema (swelling)

- Improves circulation
- Relieves lower-back pain and sciatica
- Stabilizes hormones
- Carpel tunnel
- Improves nerve pain
- Statistically reduces risk of premature labour (hypothesized to do so by reducing cortisol levels)
- Birth preparation (e.g. cervical ripening, evidenced to shorten labours)
- Natural labour induction
- Pain relief during labour
- Augmentation of contractions
- General recovery from childbirth
- Lactation and breast engorgement
- Preventing/treatment of postnatal depression

Osteopathy

Fundamentally, osteopathy recognizes the important link between body structure and body function. It uses a wide range of hands-on techniques (such as massage and stretching), plus extensive anatomical and physiological knowledge and observation, to identify somatic (bodily) dysfunction (e.g. osteopathic lesions) to treat the musculoskeletal system, and thus consequently improve health and wellbeing.

Physicians who practise as a doctor of osteopathic medicine focus on how the skeleton, muscles, joints, connective tissue (tendons and ligaments), nerves, circulation and organs all holistically function together as a unit. Manipulation of muscle tissue and bones, and mobilization of joints, are the core techniques within osteopathy, which makes it especially ideal not just for treating back, neck and pelvic pain, but also for treating headaches, asthma, middle-ear infections, and respiratory infections; and during pregnancy.

During the maternity journey, osteopathy's soft, gentle, delicate tissue massage techniques help to reduce muscle tension; and its gentle joint articulation movement manipulations help to improve nutrition in and around the joint, and increase the range of mobilization motion at specific joints; plus it assists to release and inhibit acute muscle spasms to inflamed tissues without causing further irritation.

Osteopathy has three specific maternal-wellness areas it can assist with:

Easing physical discomforts of pregnancy

- All back, neck, rib, pelvic and ligament pains, especially common lower-back discomfort (with research showing around two-thirds of pregnant women experience back pain), including sciatica
- PSD pain (pubic symphysis dysfunction)
- Headaches
- Heartburn, acid reflux, indigestion
- Constipation, diarrhoea, irritable bowel
- Haemorrhoids
- Varicosities (legs, vulva)
- Breathing issues
- Carpal tunnel
- Plantar fasciitis (foot/heel pain)
- Oedema
- Osteopath can also teach stretches, exercises and breathing techniques to assist overall pregnancy health and wellbeing

Preparing for demands of childbirth

- Fetal malposition and malpresentation
- Spine and pelvic examination to ensure bones and muscles are well aligned, to provide the optimum birth canal outlet to assist the baby's position, descent and passage
- Releasing old pelvic strains that could limit the ability for the pelvic outlet to easily open during birth
- Osteopath can also teach stretches, exercises and breathing techniques to encourage a normal birth

Helping maternal recovery during the postpartum

- General recovering from normal pregnancy postural strains and assisting return of normal alignment.
- Treating birth strains or trauma to the lower back and pelvis and supporting tissue, most commonly the coccyx or sacrum – especially after a difficult or instrumental delivery (left untreated, such unresolved strains can lead to stress incontinence, constipation, headaches and other ongoing pain and discomfort).
- Ongoing maintenance to relieve the strains from new-motherhood demands, such as from breastfeeding positions, lifting car-seats, carrying an infant on the hip.

Cranial osteopathy for newborns

The gentle art of cranial osteopathy is particularly popular for use on newborns, though it is suitable for all ages. Cranial osteopathy (aka craniosacral therapy) is a subtle form of osteopathic treatment that uses incredibly mild pressure, predominantly on the cranium (the head) though sometimes also the spine or tailbone, to encourage the release of stresses and tension throughout the body.

Because the treatment is so extremely gentle it is well suitable for babies, including very young newborns, to assist tissue moulded from the birth canal descent to release and return into its healthy state of balance, and also reduce the chance of consequential symptoms returning in the future.

In babies, cranial osteopathy can be especially effective for treating (but not limited to):

- Counteracting the effects of a difficult birth (particularly

excessive skull moulding and instrumental deliveries)
- Irritability (lessening general unsettled behaviour and increasing time of happy contentment)
- Feeding difficulties
- Improving disturbed sleep patterns
- Reducing colicky crying
- SIDE NOTE: When observing an infant receiving cranial osteopathy, it can appear as if the osteopath is almost doing "nothing", and the infant can appear as if they would purr in joy if they could purr. Also, infants often will have a long healing sleep after the session.

Reflexology

Special thanks to Dorothy Derecourt, secretary of Reflexology NZ, for her contribution to this introduction overview.

Reflexology is a natural therapy, where specific reflexes on the feet (and hands and ears) relate to corresponding specific areas of the body. By systematically working these reflexes, the body can begin to heal itself. In reflexology, treating the feet is treating the whole body.

It is an extremely therapeutic, non-invasive and relaxing therapy, during which the client remains fully clothed (sitting in a chair or lying on a massage table) and typically afterwards feels especially calm and rested.

The practice of reflexology has been recorded in historic text and images from ancient civilizations including Egypt and China. Modern reflexology has its foundations in 1917 with Dr William H Fitzgerald's "zone therapy" and subsequently with Eunice Ingham, American physiotherapist, who further researched and developed reflexology. It is the Western style of reflexology, developed by Eunice Ingham, which reflexologists mostly use today.

The benefits of reflexology are many. To name a few, reflexology reduces stress and tension, improves circulation, improves sleeping patterns and sleep quality. It can also assist in alleviating pain, assist with lymphatic function, and improve sinus congestion. It allows the body to re-balance thus promoting healing.

Conditions reflexology can assist with during the maternity journey (but not limited to):

- General pregnancy relaxation (relief of stress/anxiety)
- Mental health issues (anxiety, depression)
- Headaches relief
- Increased energy levels and reduced fatigue/tiredness/ insomnia
- Improved backache/sciatica pain
- Improved symphysis pubis (pelvic girdle) groin pain
- Reduced mood swings
- Reduced rib pain
- Heartburn, acid reflux, indigestion
- Alleviation of constipation
- Assistance with carpal tunnel syndrome
- Reducing oedema in swollen hands and feet
- It may also help with leg cramp, bleeding gums, itching skin, and over-frequency of micturition (passing urine)
- Birth preparation (e.g. cervical ripening)
- Labour acceleration and pain relief
- General recovery from childbirth
- Lactation and breast engorgement
- Prevention/treatment of postnatal depression

First trimester
Treatments are very gentle and soothing.

Second trimester
Full reflexology treatments may be given, including addressing minor ailments.

Third trimester
Ideally weekly treatments to assist with the hormonal

changes; to continue addressing any minor ailments; and to help prepare for birth.

There are also simple-to-learn techniques the reflexologist can teach the client's birthing support partner, so they can provide gentle, relaxing reflexological support throughout the pregnancy and labour.

Labour priming techniques in post-date pregnancies

If the reflexologist has attended a post-graduate maternity reflexology course, then with a pregnancy that has gone one to two weeks over the "40-week due date", there are labour-priming techniques that can be used, with awareness of the woman's midwife or obstetrician. There are also acupressure points which the trained maternity reflexologist may use as part of their priming techniques.

Neonate

Reflexology is particularly soothing for babies and may alleviate colic, gastro-oesophageal reflux, constipation, restlessness and/or irritability – and it can effectively be given to the baby by any adult. Baby reflexology is easy to learn, gentle to do, and only takes a few minutes on each foot. Any reflexologist would be able to show parents how to do this, or there is also a lot of easy-to-follow information available online. Reflexology on all babies can be particularly lovely after bath time, before bedtime, or in fact any time!

Reflex Zone Therapy (RZT)

RZT is a deeper, manipulative technique than conventional reflexology, a treatment resulting in potentially more stimulation within the body. RZT treatments tend to be shorter, or they may be incorporated into normal reflexology sessions. During the maternity journey, RZT can be especially beneficial for:

- Pregnancy or labour nausea and vomiting
- Pregnancy pelvic girdle pain.

Reiki

Developed by Mikao Usui (1865–1926), reiki translates as "universal life-force energy" and is a spiritual practice that treats physical, emotional and mental disharmony and/or disease using qi/ki (healing energy). Reiki has gained great credibility because of its amazing, often inexplicable, results. Reiki is a totally non-invasive healing technique, using a gentle-touch or non-touch methodology of relaxation and healing, working towards a balanced harmony of mind, body and soul.

Reiki is primarily used for prompt stress reduction, pain relief, and accelerated tissue healing. Reiki can also improve problem-solving abilities and enhance creativity. Because reiki is simple to learn and easy to use on yourself, family, friends, animals and plants, it is a cost-effective and immediate way of gaining enhanced health, peace of mind and wellbeing.

During a reiki session, typically a deep state of relaxation easily occurs, and with it physical, mental and emotional feelings of calmness, peace, optimism and energy renewal. Reiki is always done with the client fully clothed and is an excellent complementary therapy for cancer patients, pregnant mothers, the elderly and babies, because it is non-invasive and physically non-stimulating.

Conditions reiki can assist with during the maternity journey (but not limited to):

- General pregnancy relaxation (relief of stress/anxiety)

- Mental health Issues (anxiety, depression)
- Tiredness, fatigue
- Insomnia
- Birth preparation (e.g. cervical ripening)
- Pain relief during labour
- General recovery from childbirth
- Preventing/treatment of postnatal depression

Shiatsu

Just as the masses often struggle to understand the differences between osteopathy and chiropractic, they can also struggle to understand the differences between Chinese acupressure and Japanese shiatsu.

Unlike acupressure, which has spiritual roots in Chinese Taoism, shiatsu has spiritual roots in Indian Buddhism, however both practices are based on re-balancing qi/ki (vital energy) flow in the meridians.

In shiatsu, *tsubos* (pressure points) link the whole body, and treatment is usually full-body massage to stimulate re-balancing of the body's energy. With the client lying on a mat on the floor, the practitioner applies pressure and leans into the body, using their fingers, thumbs, palms, elbows and knees, combined with various stretching, holding and other massage manipulation techniques. It is especially wonderful as a stress-reducing treatment that balances hormones, returning the body to homeostasis.

Conditions shiatsu can assist with during the maternity journey (but not limited to):

- General pregnancy relaxation (relief of stress/anxiety)
- Mental health Issues (anxiety, depression)
- Tiredness, fatigue
- Insomnia
- Nausea and vomiting (pregnancy and labour)
- Heartburn, acid reflux, indigestion
- Constipation, diarrhoea, irritable bowel

- Haemorrhoids
- Varicosities (legs, vulva)
- Oedema
- Backache, sciatica
- Pelvic girdle pain
- Carpel tunnel
- Birth preparation (e.g. cervical ripening)
- Natural labour induction
- Pain relief during labour
- Augmentation of contractions
- Retained placenta
- General recovery from childbirth
- Lactation and breast engorgement
- Preventing/treatment of postnatal depression

Tissue Cell Salts (Mineral Therapy)

Minerals are the physical foundational building blocks of the body, upon which all other nutrients depend on for all bodily metabolic functional processes. Additionally, all digestion of nutrients such as proteins, vitamins, enzymes, amino acids and carbohydrates require minerals for absorption.

Elements also all work together as a whole – thus a shortage of even one mineral can cause nutrient imbalance inefficiencies. Consequently, even with consuming daily multi-supplement, a suboptimal cellular chemistry can result with the dietary supplement's nutrients being mal-absorbed, and consequently simply excreted by the body.

Deficiencies of mineral micro-nutrients are generally regarded as the commonest cause of dis-ease, meaning many believe you can trace practically every sickness and ailment to a mineral deficiency, which is why minerals have such a long history in treating human illness.

In the nineteenth century, Dr Wilhelm Heinrich Schuessler studied a dozen vital minerals within our cellular anatomy that act like the "workers" to assist physiology and maintain good health, and he went on to formulate easily absorbable and highly bio-available forms of these minerals called "tissue cell salts".

Tissue cell salt mineral therapy is prepared homeopathically (i.e. diluted and triturated), however it is not classical homeopathy as such. Perhaps it is best described as a "sister" to regular homeopathy, but works akin to homeopathy with its intrinsic support of homeostatic wellbeing by stimulating the body to improve regulation of its mineral absorption. Like homeopathy, tissue salts are taken sublingually (under the tongue) to absorb directly into the bloodstream (bypassing digestion) and are formulated in two versions: lactose "sugar tablets", and oral spray (using an alcohol base as the carrier preservative).

Because this mineral therapy only provides micro-doses, there is virtually no risk of adverse reactions or overdosing (logically, there exists less risk than even regular over-the-counter daily multis), which means more than one tissue salt can be taken at the same time. This also makes them completely safe for pregnant or breastfeeding women to use; safe for babies and children to take; and safe used in conjunction with all pharmaceutical drugs – though in all three circumstances we recommend patients seek a proper diagnosed treatment by a qualified tissue salt practitioner (rather than giving themselves a self-prognosis and choosing a less-effectual remedy).

Tissue salts can tend to be fast-acting, with people often able to notice subtle improvements very quickly.

Schuessler's 12 tissue salts (and their main physical actions):

- Calcium Fluoride (Calc Fluor or CF): For strength of muscles and blood vessels, connective tissue elasticity, bones, enamel, and can support depression caused by extreme stress.
- Calcium Phosphate (Calc Phos or CP): The "cell builder" for bone, connective tissue, blood, and teeth; and great for kids' growing pains.
- Calcium Sulphate (Calc Sulph or CS): A "blood cleanser"

and purifier, which also helps to clear suppuration (reduce pus). Especially beneficial for liver, blood, and skin conditions.

- Iron Phosphate (Ferrum Phos or IP): Reduces swelling and pain (the first stage of inflammation) by helping the formation of red blood corpuscles and strengthens blood vessels. Ideal for first aid, colds, nose bleeds, and fever.
- Potassium Chloride (Kali Mur or PC): A "decongestant" anti-inflammatory, which is essential for blood, muscles and mucous membranes. Also for the second stage of head colds with its inflammatory swollen glands and earaches.
- Potassium Phosphate (Kali Phos or PP): A "nerve nutrient" so perfect for anxiety, brain fog, bedwetting, and insomnia.
- Potassium Sulphate (Kali Sulph or PS): The "cell-transport oxygenator", which can clear third-stage inflammation such as stubborn mucous and skin conditions.
- Magnesium Phosphate (Mag Phos or MP): Ideal for muscles and nerves, this remedy is an antispasmodic natural pain reliever of cramps, tension, spasms, stress-related pain headaches, and menstrual cramps.
- Sodium Chloride (Nat Mur or SC): The "fluid balancer" that distributes salts, supports mucous membranes, relieves heavy emotions, and benefits dry skin, mucous membranes, and hay fever.
- Sodium Phosphate (Nat Phos or SP): A natural antacid (metabolic acid remover) that works like a system neutralizer, and stress reliever. Great for arthritis, stiffness, and digestive complaints.
- Sodium Sulphate (Nat Sulph or SS): The "detoxifier"

diuretic and liver decongestant. A cleanser that is also ideal for water retention and liver issues.

- Silicea (Silica or S): The "calcium-organizer" that strengthens tissue (e.g. connective, bones, teeth). Ideal for healthy hair, nails and skin, plus also clears suppuration and foreign matter from the body. Great for the not-so-young!

Traditional Chinese Medicine (TCM)

Rooted in ancient medical texts, traditional Chinese medicine is more than 3500 years old and is based on many interconnected philosophies, with central ideas being:

- YIN AND YANG (cosmological unity of opposites): *yin* being dark, cold, solid (digestion, bladder, oestrogen, progesterone, pregnancy, postpartum); *yang* being bright, warm, positive (liver, heart, spleen, lungs, kidney, testosterone, oxytocin, developing fetus, labour)
- QI/CH'I (life-force energy vitality) and the body's meridians (flow of qi/ch'i energy-pathway channels)
- WUXING: Five Elements or Five Phases (water, metal, earth, wood and fire).

TCM observes that human bodily processes interact with, and are interrelated to, the universal environment. TCM regards *health* as the *harmonious* interaction of all these entities and the outside world, and it regards *ill-health* as the *disharmony* of such interactions.

Practitioners recognize the signs of imbalance or disharmony in order to diagnose, prevent and treat illness and disease, believing that optimum health results from living harmoniously. TCM physicians diagnose wellness and disease using multiple observations, including the patient's sleep habits, pulse and appearance of their tongue, skin and eyes.

Western medicine focuses mainly on treating disease. But

like so many Asian and indigenous wellness philosophies, TCM looks holistically at your entire wellbeing – physically, mentally, emotionally, spiritually. Western medicine tends to view the body akin to a vehicle that has different systems that need concrete logical inputs and outputs, whereas TCM is based on balance, harmony, and energy.

TCM believes that when you harmoniously balance the yin and yang flow of qi, then you feel healthy and well. But when qi is out of harmonious balance, then you feel unhealthy and unwell.

TCM is mainstream medicine in China and Taiwan, and its therapies include:

- Herbal formulas
- Acupuncture
- Moxibustion (the burning of 'moxa' or mugwort herb)
- Cupping therapy
- Gua sha ('scraping' to skin to increase circulation)
- Die-da ('bonesetter' joint manipulation)
- Tui na (bodywork massage)
- Qigong (exercise)
- Tai chi (martial art)
- Feng shui (environmental energy)
- Dietary therapy
- Chinese astrology

TCM is particularly useful for long-term treatment of chronic conditions, cravings, and for general health and wellbeing. In China, TCM uses at least 500 herbs with more than 400 patented herbal remedies. Recipes that are thousands of years old are still used today – though not all medicines are available internationally.

In the 1950s, the Chinese government began promoting a standardized form of TCM, integrating it with the modern medical knowledge on anatomy and physiology. And as it does globally, Big Pharma research continues to explore the potential within TCM herbalism for creating new patentable synthetic drug molecules based on traditional remedies.

In TCM the health of both parents at conception impacts the quality (strength, weaknesses) of the child's constitution, and the point that the pregnant mother is both a physical and spiritual "vessel" into which the growing fetus's health and intelligence is impacted by every aspect of the mother's health – and today's current cutting-edge epigenetics is certainly beginning to scientifically confirm these ancient theories.

TCM believes the baby inherits a quantity and quality of "inborn qi" from its parents (and respective ancestors) that forms its "energy foundation", which is greatly influenced not just by the mother's pregnancy wellbeing, but also by the baby's non-traumatic vs traumatic experience of the birth delivery. (Midwives and holistic healers have been preaching this mandate from time immemorial!)

TCM pregnancy guidelines

In TCM, the goal is to gift the child for their lifetime the foundation of good health from a strong constitutional energy of body-mind-spirit. This is achieved by the pregnant mother following these directives:

- Reduce stress including reducing workload*
- Nap during the day, and retire early at night
- Avoid caffeine, alcohol, smoking and eating raw or cold foods (i.e. no salads)
- Eat fresh, healthy, organic, easily-digested in-season fruits and vegetables, served cooked and warm
- Increase fish consumption
- There are also many types of TCM teas that are safe in pregnancy and can support the body's qi balance
- Practise qigong meditative exercise stretches
- Listen to classical music, sending peaceful messages to your baby
- Receive soft and gentle *tui na* massage
- Medicinal herbs in low doses prescribed professionally can also be especially helpful with pregnancy wellness
- Regularly visit an acupuncturist to assess energy levels
- Reduce exposure of environmental toxins including use of cellphones and wireless devices
- The classical herbal formula *Bu-Zhong-Yi-Qi-Tang* is very safe for pregnancy, and used for raising qi, and to prevent recurring miscarriages as well as for treating placenta previa.

Author Comment

Westernized women (particularly European) can socially struggle terribly within modern society to feel they have permission to follow this instruction. There exists a warped mentality around the robust hardiness of pregnant women, believing they should "be at the gym several times a week, and work up until 37 weeks", which is insanity.

For my entire career as a case-loading midwife I have

preached to my clients to *work part-time from 28 weeks, and not working from 32 weeks* – and even earlier for women with pre-existing medical complexities or pregnancies experiencing obstetric complications. I am *convinced* following those strategies leads to less pregnancy problems developing, leading to less inductions being indicated, leading to less epidural-oxytocin labours, resulting in way more normal births, and high fully-exclusive breastfeeding rates, and virtually no maternal postnatal depression. (Interestingly, during Covid-19 lockdowns, NICU units around the world became extraordinarily quiet, due to the substantially reduced amounts of pre-term labours of premature babies … and in my opinion this was directly because most expectant women were chilling at home, instead of going to work.)

To avoid the *Cascade of Intervention*, protecting the *Cascade of Normalcy* begins in pregnancy!

TCM post-pregnancy guidelines

It is normal for a woman to lose up to 500 ml or 1 pint of blood after birth, and it is not uncommon for women to lose double that. In TCM, blood and qi are directly linked (i.e. blood loss is also qi loss). This, it is believed, makes the woman weakened and very vulnerable, especially to catching cold, even in summer (with her qi loss making it easier for cold to penetrate her meridians), which leads to muscle, joint and/or nerve pain.

TCM also views childbirth like a "gateway door" into a potentially enhanced state of future health and wellbeing. TCM believes that after childbirth, a woman's body and mind are very open, creating a great opportunity for her to be strengthened ... thus making it a time she should be very well cared for especially during the first month called *zuo yuezi* (translates to "sitting out a month") when the new mother should relax and do as little as possible (and is traditionally looked after by her mother-in-law).

General postpartum TCM to-do list:

- Soft and gentle *tui na* massage
- Avoid all things cold: cold beverages, cold uncooked food, cold water, air-conditioning
- Avoid ice packs[*]
- Rest, rest, rest
- Eat plenty of fresh, healthy, organic fruits, vegetables and fish, served cooked and warm
- Take classical herbal formula supplements prescribed by TCM practitioner to support and rebuild blood and qi, and help stabilize emotions.

Author Comment

However, ice packs on a sore, sutured perineum in the first 24 hours do feel wonderful, as do refrigerated hydrogel disc pads on sore, traumatized nipples.

Western Herbal Medicine

Let food be our medicine and medicine be our food.

Hippocrates, Greek physician (468–377 BCE)

With its intimate connection with Gaia (Mother Earth), *herbal medicine* globally is quite literally human history's oldest healing therapies for ailments, and its accumulated knowledge of the curative values of plants (flowers, leaves, fruit, bark and roots) has been passed from generation to generation for thousands of years. Traditionally all over the planet, native societies would often have the male shaman responsible for the moral wellbeing of their villagers, and a female healer-midwife responsible for the physical wellbeing of their community.

In ancient Europe, traditional Western herbal medicine mostly evolved from the Greeks who were strongly influenced by the Middle Eastern civilizations, especially Egypt. The Greek god Asclepius was the god of healing disease; and his daughter Hygieia was the healthy-lifestyle goddess watching over her people (thus today's word "hygiene" meaning free from bacteria); and her sister Panacea was believed to possess omnipotent healing powers (with "panacea" today meaning cure-all).

The Greeks believed "energy" is the positive spiritual life-force, and "matter" is the opposing negative force – with combining the two being regarded as creating the Four Elements, being fire, water, earth, air ... thus creating *Life!*

With the Romans invading Celtic Britain (and Celtic France and Germany), the indigenous Druidic healing practices became ostracized, however "underground" they remained strongly influential until the late 1900s – even surviving through the thousand years of Western Europe's Dark Ages, a time when God and astrology was strongly believed to be the powers influencing all sickness.

Three thousand years ago the "father of medicine" Hippocrates (where the doctors' Hippocratic Oath stems from) infamously taught, *"It is more important to know what kind of person has a disease, than to know what kind of disease a person has"* – a philosophy that remains fundamental today to all modalities of holistic Eastern healing, and continues to remain fundamentally irrelevant to most of modern Western medicine … *oh such stubborn blindness continuing for so long. Sigh!*

Perhaps the most influential Western physician of all lived just over 2000 years ago, Galen, whose medical theories were regarded as fact throughout Europe for several hundred years thereafter, and even remained required medical reading until only a few hundred years ago.

In fact, European history is teeming with famous herbal healer physicians and books, including *De Materia Medica* ("The Medical Material"), which became Europe's main medical text for hundreds of years.

Eventually Western medicine evolved to be defined as the *Four Cardinal Humours* ("hinge fluids") of Hot, Cold, Wet and Dry; that result in the *Four Liquid Humours* (yellow bile, black bile, blood and phlegm); which are all influenced by the *Four Personality Temperaments* (choleric, melancholic, sanguine and phlegmatic).

At the same time as Europe's Dark Ages, Islamic Arabian countries were enjoying an intellectual pinnacle, and a thousand years ago they solidified Galen's hypotheses of using positive qualities of a plant to correct negative characteristics of a disease (which happens to also still be today's like-cure-like principles of both homeopathy and vaccine inoculations).

After the Dark Ages, European Benedictine monks began to move away from alchemist tonics to teaching healing wellness, with a separation of the *church* (spiritual-mind disease) and *medicine* (physical-body ailments) ... though village folk-medicine remained influenced by the mystical and magical for hundreds of years.

Five hundred years ago, as Europe moved into the Renaissance period, healing was also rebirthed to focus on empirical (evidence-based) models of allopathic (science-based) medicine. The physical body got termed the "horizontal axis", and life-force energy got termed the "vertical axis", with perfect health being the centre of the mid-point crossover. At the same time in Britain, disputes between traditional botanical healers and modern alchemical therapists resulted in a charter protecting herbalists' rights.

A century later in the early 1600s, English botanist, herbalist and physician Nicholas Culpeper translated the *London Pharmacopoeia* from Latin to English, making it available for the first time beyond just academic scholars. Then in the mid-1600s he published *The Complete Herbal* discourse of the cures to all disorders, which is still in print today.

In the late 1700s the first herb (foxglove) was lost from herbalists for treating 'dropsy' (cardiac oedema), when English botanist William Withering isolated its glycosides, changing the foxglove plant from being an ancient village-alchemist medicinal herb to becoming the pharmaceutical drug digoxin, to thereafter be prescribed only by "licensed practitioners". This continues today in pharmacology with hundreds of drugs derived from plants, purloined by modern medicine, for example to name just a few: atropine, benzyl benzoate, bromelain, codeine, digoxin, morphine, pseudoephedrine.

These days, Western medical herbalists are able to routinely access the highest quality of ethically-sourced plant extracts in multiple herbal forms (liquids, tablets, powders and teas), which are routinely fantastic alternatives to modern conventional meds, particularly anti-inflammatories, and analgesics (pain relievers), plus the herbal remedies undergo stringent quality testing for purity and strength – and are typically devoid of the plethora of unpleasant adverse-reaction side-effects that are commonplace to the synthetic (royalty-income-producing) equivalent within pharmaceutical drugs.

Qualified WMH practitioners also have access to supplements with stronger bio-availability, which aren't available as OTCs (over-the-counters). Today, Western herbal medicines routinely also include Native American herbs adopted by European American pioneers, such as echinacea, black cohosh, cranberry and American ginseng.

Collectively, Western medical herbalism can be extremely effective to help treat and help prevent many illnesses, with it being especially popular for stress-tension musculoskeletal-related conditions, and general health wellness support, including:

- Arthritis and joint pain
- General pain
- Swelling
- Muscle tension and cramps
- Injury recovery
- Improving sleep issues
- Digestion
- Respiratory system
- Circulation
- Immune system
- Endocrine system
- Nervous system processes
- Toxin/waste removal
- Topical skin healing

Conditions WHM can assist with during the maternity journey (but not limited to):

- Mental health (e.g. depression, anxiety)
- Tiredness, fatigue, insomnia
- Nausea and vomiting during pregnancy and labour
- Haemorrhoids
- Varicosities (legs, vulva)
- Oedema
- Natural labour induction (prescribed by qualified herbalist)
- Wound healing and Infection
- General recovery from birth
- Lactation

Modern *Big Pharma* continues to research plant medicinal qualities to find the next useful natural molecule they can successfully facsimile into a unique synthetic molecule, to then deliver "standardized set doses" *and* earn *big* drug royalties. (NB: Royalties cannot be earned on any molecules that naturally occur in nature.)

Many believe – *moi included* – that the ultimate cure to all the disease on the planet ultimately resides within all plants on this planet ... we just haven't yet discovered all the "what-cures-what".

Points to Note

SPECIAL NOTE 1: Overviews Only

All of the prior information is summarized introductions only and should never be regarded as medical guidelines.

That especially relates to women and babies regarded as high risk, who are best to seek naturopathic advice from qualified practitioners – in conjunction with their obstetric consultations – rather than self-diagnosing and purchasing online/over-the-counter traditional holistic medicines.

This particularly relates to, but is not limited to:

- Anticoagulant disease or meds
- Cardiac disease
- Diabetes mellitus
- Epilepsy
- Hypertension, especially pre-elampsic toxaemia
- Liver disease
- Respiratory conditions (e.g. asthma)
- Skin conditions (e.g. eczema, psoriasis)
- Twin/triplet pregnancy
- Vaginal bleeding or placental issues
- Premature pre-term neonates

SPECIAL NOTE 2: Safe and Unsafe Summary

Regarding specific **essential oils** and especially **herbal medicines**, there does exist substantial conflicting information around what are and aren't contraindicated (considered unsafe) during pregnancy, labour and breastfeeding. It is extremely easy to find differing opinions. And for that reason, I do recommend women always consult with a qualified naturopathic health professional, be it aromatherapy, Ayurvedic herbal medicine, traditional Chinese medicine, or Western herbal medicine.

In general, **Bach's flower essence** remedies, **homeopathy** remedies and **tissue salts** are very safe for women to self-diagnose and self-treat during their maternity journey. They are also wonderful first-cab-off-the-rank healing treatments for parents to confidently use initially with their babies and children, especially for the mild–moderate issues. And to, of course, seek a professional medical opinion should the condition be severe, continuing or worsening. Additionally, these three holistic modalities are excellent restorative remedies to assist a baby or child to recovery *after* an illness, to assist their body to return to its natural homeostatic equilibrium physically, mentally and emotionally.

Critical Points to Note

When referring to next sections in this book, rational common sense must always prevail!

Information on the following pages does *not* replace historic advice of care-plan management and does *not* replace usual appropriate intervention of medical actions by the midwife, obstetrician or paediatrician.

This information is designed as an additional complement to standard midwifery education and routine obstetric protocols.

A naturopathic remedy may completely resolve the situation, or simply act as a first-aid measure to buy time, or be an assisting boost to emergency procedures.

The author can take *no* responsibility for the reader's interpretation and use of any or all of this information. It is provided as an introductory guide to perinatal integrative medicine.

Rational commonsense must always prevail!

What the following pages do and don't contain

These chapters don't contain *all* potential integrative maternity healthcare remedies; they intentionally provide simply an overview as a general handbook guideline of the most well-recognized therapies for the commonest and easily identifiable conditions.

As a health professional, you can confidently pass this advice to your clients, *at your discretion*, because many of the listed remedies are naturopathic and homeopathic OTC therapies that do not require a qualified practitioner prescription. Therefore, you are simply assisting your client to sift through the plethora of Dr Google options to improve their odds of finding the right remedy for their condition to effect prompt healing.

The Antepartum (Pregnancy)

Pre-conception

Today there exists an exponentially growing amount of knowledge around the importance of the pre-conception period, particularly the immediate three months prior to fertilization. Science is discovering, conclusively, the benefits of good pre-conception health and how this impacts not only the quality of the egg and sperm, but also the beneficial effects this can have on the health of the developing fetus.

Collectively the emerging sciences, especially Epigenetics, is nothing less than mind-blowing. The preparation (or lack of preparation) couples apply before conception can set their child up for the rest of their life. And ultimately influences their child's health as an adult.

In general terms the recommended supplement fundamental basics are designed to provide essential nutrients needed before pregnancy for the potential fetus, along with enhancing glandular and libido balance for both the mother and the father.

Simplest overview of pre-conception nutrition:

FOR HER: A quality women's multi to provide the complete array of vitamins and minerals essential to the support of both mother and baby during preconception and pregnancy, to enrich her nutrient supplies particularly of folic acid, calcium, iodine, and magnesium. Plus, a non-constipating form of iron to help ensure complete nutritional support.

FOR HIM: Many men have low-quality sperm without

realizing. Free radical damage is a major contributor to affecting sperm quality and health, often resulting in fertility issues in men. An antioxidant with zinc and selenium especially, can play a vital role in improving sperm quality and motility.

FOR THEM: A boost to the glandular system to assist with libido for both him and her, such as the hormone-free extract from the Peruvian root *maca*, with its glandular-balancing effect, boosting sexual function and enhancing fertility.

Routine Pregnancy Care

With general pregnancy wellness investment, the guideline can be incredibly straightforward:

- *A good daily multi and omega-3 DHA.*
- *Plus probiotics, calcium and iron supplementation.*

Firstly, choosing a great-quality pregnancy multi specifically formulated to contain essential nutrients such as folic acid and iodine, as well as iron, calcium and vitamin D – along with all the most important fundamental nutritional support for all pregnant women. These nutrients support the growth and development of the fetus, while the addition of vitamin B6 may help to manage symptoms of morning sickness. *However, it is a general consensus amongst naturopaths that the supply of calcium and iron contained in OTC 'preggy dailies' is suboptimal.*

NB: The most expensive and/or the most advertised does not always equate with best value or best quality. Some multi manufacturers simply have larger advertising budgets than others! I recommend getting advice from the naturopath at a local health shop rather than asking the pharmacist at a local drug store.

Secondly, we already know about the importance of omega-3 oil for healthy brain *function*, but this essential DHA fatty acid at an optimum level is even more important for healthy brain *growth*. A high-quality supplement helps to maintain the mother's stores, and to also provide DHA for the baby's healthy brain, eye, cellular membrane and central nervous system development.

Thirdly, all mothers of course want a healthy baby, but they are typically also hopeful to be blessed with a calm content baby too. In my extensive experience of observation, by providing a rich supply of the soothing mineral Calcium and Magnesium, with their co-factors many mothers specifically comment later about how their baby is "the most easy to please and chilled out of their whole prenatal group". Apart from a diet really high in such nutrients (a pregnant woman needs 1500–1800mg of calcium every day), a highly absorbable mineral supplement can be an effective way to help do this.

Finally, as in optional extra: It is not uncommon to experience thrush or a urinary tract infection (UTI) during pregnancy, even if for women who have not been prone to these before. Science has realized the importance of consuming certain probiotics to support the immune system of beneficial bacteria while pregnant, to help prevent these problems by helping the gut health's inner bacterial balance, as well as help in the prevention of skin problems like eczema in baby.

Common Discomforts of Pregnancy

Bacterial Vaginosis (vaginal infection)

HERBALISM/NUTRITION/HOMEOPATHY

- Increase garlic in the diet. Also finely chop garlic, steep it in water, then douche with it
- Probiotic supplement
- Avoid carbohydrate sugars
- See nutritionist or naturopath if persists/recurrent
- Homeopathy: Sepia

Biliary Colic (Gallstone/gallbladder attack)

Main Homeopathic remedy: Chelidonium majus

Breast Pain

Painful discomfort from mammogenesis-II and lactogenesis: Homeopathy: Conium mac or Bryonia.

Carpal Tunnel Syndrome

NATUROPATHY/NUTRITION

- Many potentially contributory reasons, particularly high uric acid (watch the diet)
- Add magnesium (especially for stiff joints)
- Consider adding a high-strength omega-3 supplement
- Magnesium oil/cream applied topically

- (Limited with herbs as they are bile producers.)

ESSENTIAL OILS

- Frankincense, marjoram, lemongrass, oregano and cypress
- A few drops of each, or individually, diluted in tablespoon fractionated coconut oil and applied to wrists

HOMEOPATHY

- General remedy: Blend of Arnica, Bellis, Ruta, Hypericum and Mag sulph. Take 2 drops under the tongue, 3–4 times a day or as required. And/or add 4–6 drops in 300ml of warm water, shake, and sip throughout the day.
- Soreness/weakness in the fingers is dominant or lacking strength to grip things: Arnica
- Computer-related strained ligaments: Ruta
- Injury-related: Arnica
- Inflamed carpel tendons compressing the median nerve: Bellis and Ruta
- Strained ligaments and pain to the bone: Bellis and Ruta
- Tingling sensation in the fingers (or thumb and fingers): Hypericum
- Sensation of something crawling on the fingers: Hypericum
- Pain, numbness and a tingling sensation in the thumb and fingers: Bellis and Ruta
- To loosen joints: Mag sulph

Chloasma (mask of pregnancy)

Main Homeopathic remedy: Sepia

Colds and Flu

ESSENTIAL OIL

- Melaleuca rubbed on chest
- Consider a therapist-created protective or respiratory blend on chest

HOMEOPATHY FOR COMMON COLD

- General remedy: Blend of Antimonium tart, Aconite, Gelsemium, Hepar sulph and Hypericum. Take 2 drops under the tongue, 3–4 times a day or as required. And/or add 4–6 drops in 300ml of warm water, shake, and sip throughout the day.
- Sudden exposure to cold weather: Aconite
- Chesty cough: Antimonium tart
- Sore throat, nerve pains, discomfort: Hypericum
- Irritable coughing episodes: Hepar sulph
- Weakness and fever: Gelsemium

INFLUENZA-LIKE ILLNESS

- Review diet, micronutrients, boost immune system and consult with naturopath/homeopath
- (With pyrexia fever, absolutely seek a medical consultation – true Influenza is serious in pregnancy.)

Constipation

Potential causes include tension (holding on), laziness (need fibre), or not going then it's loose. Many potential remedies but check diet first.

Many useful remedies depending on specific symptoms. Consult with herbalist. Examples:

- Change diet (reduce carbohydrates and refined food)
- Add lemon, ginger and honey (ginger stimulates peristalsis)
- Take an "inner health" supplement
- Make a salad of raw grated beetroot, carrot and swede, with a lemon and oil dressing (bowel movement will resemble rectal bleeding due to the beetroot)
- Lemon essential oil diluted in tablespoon fractionated coconut oil and applied to the abdomen
- If condition is chronic, consult with qualified naturopath

HOMEOPATHY

Many useful remedies – following are some examples – worth consulting with homeopath.

- Main remedies: Nux vomia and Sepia
- No bowel movement at all: Opium
- Fear of bowel movement: Aconite
- 'Holding on' tendency: Natrum mur
- Lack of 'feeling the need' (typically post-epidural or traumatic delivery): Opium
- Recovering from shock: Aconite
- Impatience to 'complete the job': Nux vomica

- Third-trimester constipation: Collinsonia

Diarrhoea

HERBALISM/NUTRITION

- Diarrhoea is usually caused by a viral, parasitic or bacterial infection, and rehydration is the first port of call. Red raspberry also useful. (Can't use slippery elm in pregnancy before 35 weeks.) Probiotic strain *L. reuteri* specific remedy for diarrhoea. Potatoes and rice absorb extra fluid.
- High-sugar drink, e.g. Coca-Cola (radical but true: insulin elevates → urine increases → stools harden)
- Consuming potatoes/rice (absorb extra fluid)
- If chronic, see a naturopath, herbalist or homeopath

ESSENTIAL OILS

- Ginger and Geranium applied topically diluted in fractionated coconut oil
- Consider a therapist's digestion blend

HOMEOPATHY

Way too many potential remedies depending on the complete big picture. Examples:

- "Splatters everywhere" diarrhoea: Croton tig
- From bad food (or from a constipation-causing diet): Arsenicum alb
- Watery black/yellow acrid stools: Arsenicum alb
- Painless watery stools: China
- Frequent watery stools and gripping pain: China

- From the use of antibiotics: Nitricum acidum

Dyspnea (mild shortness of breath)

Main Homeopathic remedies: Calc carb and Carb veg

Emotions (Intense)

HOMEOPATHY

As well as Bach's flower essences (such as *Rescue Remedy*) taking the edge off unproductive or debilitating emotions, this is where homeopathy can reign supreme, allowing the person to feel renewed sensations of happy contentment.

- General anxiety: Aconite, Gelsemium, Arsenicum alb
- Ambitious (dislike being contradicted): Nux vomica
- Compulsive (fastidious in nature): Nux vomica
- Enjoyed stimulants (e.g. coffee, alcohol) pre-pregnancy: Nux vomica
- Multip indifferent with pregnancy: Sepia
- Weepy and needy: Pulsatilla
- Stubborn and angry: Pulsatilla
- Peevish and easily offended: Capsicum
- Holding on to discord: Natrum mur
- Anger in general, and anger at husband and family relatives: Sepia
- Anxiety about money: Arsenicum alb
- Anxiety about becoming a mother: Natrum mur
- Anxiety about losing friends: Pulsatilla

Epistaxis (nosebleeds)

Main Homeopathic remedy: Phos

Exhaustion/Fatigue

HERBALISM

First, get stored-iron blood-check, especially beyond 32 weeks. (Preferably have a baseline Ferritin with booking bloods to immediately address unknown pre-existing chronic Iron anaemia before it becomes more acute in pregnancy.)

Second, take a superior iron supplement, combined with homeopathic Ferrum phos to assist oxygen transportation.

If persists, see a naturopath and acupuncturist.

ESSENTIAL OILS

1–2 drops thyme oil diluted in tablespoon fractionated coconut oil and applied to the feet/body, and/or diffused. Consider a therapist's serenity blend to bring a sense of calm.

NUTRITION

- Consume a "Dr Gundry" diet (Google it) – the worst thing for tiredness is sugar – so avoid refined foods including sugars, pasta, noodles, rice
- Increase dietary polyphenols (e.g. olive oil, currants, dark berries, dark chocolate, flaxseed meal)
- Eat foods that boost energy levels, especially blueberries, raspberries, strawberries and apples
- Eat foods high in magnesium, especially cashews, almonds and hazelnuts. They assist to convert sugar to

energy, and are filled with fibre to keep blood-sugar levels stable. Recommend clients keep a bag of mixed nuts on hand.

- Protein balances blood-sugar levels and staves off hunger
- Cardamom increases energy and promotes blood flow by expanding the small blood vessels
- Sauerkraut (fermented cabbage) helps maintain energy. It is also high in probiotics that help the gut break down foods (so the body works less to digest and saves energy)
- Asparagus is high in B vitamins which support energy levels, assisting to turn carbohydrates into glucose because of containing generous blood-sugar-stabilizing fibre – especially good at lunchtime to boost energy
- Adding lemon to water transforms regular water into a natural energy drink packed with electrolytes

HOMEOPATHY

- Extreme exhaustion: Arsenicum alb
- Mental fatigue: Phosphoric acid
- Physical exhaustion: Fluoric acid
- From loss of body fluids (e.g. postpartum haemorrhage): China
- General exhaustion remedy: Blend of Fluoric acid, Phosphoric acid, Kali phos and China. Take 2 drops under the tongue, 3–4 times a day or as required. And/or add 4–6 drops in 300ml of warm water, shake, and sip throughout the day. (Also suitable for childbirth and postpartum.)
- Rescue Remedy also useful.

Gingivitis (bleeding gums)

Main Homeopathic remedy: Phos

Group B Strep

Common bacterium found in the vagina, bladder or bowel of about one in five women.

Antibiotics recommended during active labour to inhibit transfer to the baby.

HERBALISM/NUTRITION

- Increase garlic in the diet
- Finely chop garlic, steep it in water, then douche vagina
- See naturopath or herbalist if persistent/recurrent

Haemorrhoids

Many causations exist that exacerbate the existence of this condition, including too many carbohydrates and insulin resistance.

NATUROPATHY

- Consume an inner-health supplement, Tissue-Salt Combination-G.
- Use a natural product such as Aesculus and Hamamelis haemorrhoid suppositories, or Presto Gel haemorrhoid treatment.
- If persists, see naturopath or herbalist.

ESSENTIAL OIL

Blend 1–2 drops cypress diluted in tablespoon fractionated coconut oil, and apply to the haemorrhoids using a rectal syringe.

HOMEOPATHY

- From trauma to area: Simillimum's Trauma mix
- Internal and painful piles: Nux vomica
- Changeable symptoms: Pulsatilla
- Large blue and itchy piles: Carbo veg
- Piles desiring warmth as pain relief: Arsenicum alb
- General blend: Aesculus, Hypericum, Bellis and Hamamelis. Apply 2–4 drops directly onto haemorrhoid. And/or put 4–6 drops in cup of warm water, soak a cloth, and apply to haemorrhoids for at least one hour.

Hayfever

HOMEOPATHY: Chrome alum

NUTRITION

- Quercetin – antihistamine flavonoid (found in berries, parsley, onions and peppers)
- Biotin – vitamin B helps health of mucous membranes (found in offal, fish, egg yolks, avocados, green leafy veg)
- Herbal teas – natural antihistamine qualities of green tea, chamomile, elderflower, ginger, peppermint and anise
- Probiotics – multi-strain supplement, plus sauerkraut, bone broths, gelatine, natural and kefir yoghurt
- Local honey – good evidence shows this exposure to the local pollen assists
- Garlic – dietary and supplement, assists to block

histamine production

- Vitamin D deficiency – is linked to allergy and autoimmune diseases, so sunlight and a daily multi with vitamin D could assist

Headaches (minor)

Always check blood pressure to rule out pre-exclamsic toxaemia.

NATUROPATHY/NUTRITION

- Check iron levels and drink more water (80 per cent are caused by dehydration)
- Schuessler Tissue Salt No. 9 Nat Mur combined with homeopathic Nat mur for healthy fluid-balance water distribution
- If persists see osteopath and naturopath – *and* report to midwife/obstetrician for a blood pressure check

ESSENTIAL OIL

- Apply topically or diffuse: Cardamom
- Consider a therapist's tension blend

HOMEOPATHY

- Main remedies: Belladonna, Lac defloratum, Cham, Natrum sulph, Nux vomica and Pulsatilla
- Early pregnancy with no reason (fluid imbalance): Natrum mur
- Left-sided: Sepia
- From fluid imbalance: Calc phos
- Migraine: Calc phos

- If persists, see homeopath for constitutional case by case

Hypersalivation

Main Homeopathic remedies: Pulsatilla and Ipecac

Indigestion Heartburn

HERBALISM/NUTRITION

- Reduce carbs (they are the cause of most reflux)
- Take inner-health supplement
- Chlorophyll liquid (between meals)
- Schuessler Tissue Salt No. 10 Nat Phos (the natural antacid acid-neutraliser)
- 1–2 drops lemon essential oil diluted in tablespoon fractionated coconut oil and applied to the chest. Can also be diffused.
- If persists chronically, see naturopath

HOMEOPATHY

- Main heartburn remedies: Arsenicum alb, Lycopodium, Natrum mur and Natrum phos
- Main indigestion remedies: Cocculus, Nux vomica, Pulsatilla and Sepia
- From overindulgence: Nux vomica
- With flatulence from vegetables (especially for vegetarians when also gassy): Carbo veg
- Without acid feeling: Pulsatilla or Capsicum
- With mild acid feeling: Calc carb
- With burning-acid feeling: Calc sulph or Capsicum

- With belly feeling bloated: Natrum mur (also aids digestion)
- General blend: Nux vomica, Carbo veg, Natrum sulph, Calcarea phos and Dioscorea to help assimilate and digest food, support bowel peristalsis, reduce burning/cramping sensation discomfort, eliminate gas and constipation.

Insomnia (sleeping difficulties)

Common diagnosed causes: working too intensely, and overwhelmed with tasks and deadlines. Common undiagnosed cause: gut unhappiness.

HERBALISM/NUTRITION

- Useful supplements include calcium-magnesium mineral powder. Chamomile tea
- Plus, Schuessler Tissue Salt No. 6 Kali Phos (nerve nutrient) combined with homeopathic Kali phos (the natural tranquilliser)
- Useful relaxation therapies include a bath, massage, deep-breathing techniques, and meditation to balance the mind and remove negativity
- If persists see acupuncturist, herbalist, naturopath. (Consider faecal transplant.)

ESSENTIAL OILS

Lavender, wild orange, roman chamomile and spikenard.

HOMEOPATHY FOR SLEEPLESSNESS

- Main remedies: Coffea, Nux vom and Rhus tox

- With general fear: Aconite
- With excitement: Arsenicum alb
- With fears about health of the baby or herself:
  Arsenicum alb
- From overwork/mind racing/too many thoughts: Nux
  vomica
- From grief or worries about relationships or wanting to
  make things perfect: Ignatia
- From feelings about being a good mother/holding on to
  old grievances: Natrum mur
- From overwork, or anger with family/husband: Sepia
- From feeling bruises/bed feeling too hard: Arnica
- *Many* more remedies exist for other conditions
- General blend: Nux vomica, Coffea, Ignatia, Natrum mur,
  Ruta and Arnica.
- If repeatedly waking at certain times each overnight: see
  classical homeopath for constitutional consultation.

Iron Anaemia (Iron Depletion)

Depleted iron stores in pregnancy is *extremely* common, and
consistently poorly diagnosed. The woman can feel fatigued,
emotionally erratic, breathless, and/or unable to focus – but
she will oftentimes assume she is feeling tired just because
she is pregnant. The key is: prevention. Recommendation
is a ferritin baseline check with booking bloods, repeated
at 24–26 weeks, and potentially again at 32–33 weeks if
symptomatic.

HERBALISM/NUTRITION

- Essential: Take a superior quality highly-absorbable iron
  supplement that contains all the important co-factors to
  enhance absorption. Plus, Schuessler Tissue Salt No. 4

Ferr Phos (the "first aid" oxygen transporter).
- Spirulina combo that features a rich concentration of nutrients, large dandelion, and nettle tea.
- If Hb < 90 g/l (and not responding to treatment) seek a medical consultation, as well as dietary advice, organic supplements, acupuncture consult and homeopathy consult.

HOMEOPATHY

Homeopathy can help with anaemia, especially for women who poorly absorb dietary iron.

- Main remedy (aids absorption and gives natural boost of oxygen): Ferrum phos
- Woman who looks healthy but abdomen is pale: Ferrum met
- Chronic pre-existing anaemia from menorrhagia: Ferrum met
- Haemorrhage-induced anaemia: China
- Anaemia with grief: Natrum mur
- Anaemia with desire to eat chalk/paper/soil: Nitric acid
- Anaemia with weakness/exhaustion: Ferrum phos
- Anaemia with extreme fatigue/fainting: Aletris farinosa
- Anaemia with vertigo, pulsating headaches or tinnitus: Ferrum met
- Anaemia with dyspnoea/palpitations: Ferrum met
- Weak with paleness, and frequent false flushing appearance from excitement (flushed face but pale, cold body): Ferrum met
- General blend of Ferrum phos, Aletris farinosa, China and Ferrum met. Take 2 drops under the tongue 3–4 times a day. And/or 4–6 drops shaken in a cup of warm water and sipped throughout the day.

Joint Stiffness

Main Homeopathic remedy: Rhus tox

Leg Cramps

HERBALISM/NUTRITION

- Diet rich in magnesium especially (plus calcium, zinc, sodium and potassium)
- To prevent leg cramps, three times a day lean against the wall with feet flat on the floor

HOMEOPATHY

- Main remedies: Mag phos (for slender build) and Calc phos (for larger build)
- Other go-to remedies: Verat alb, Nux vomica or Ledum
- General blend of Mag sulph, Zinc and Natrum mur. Take 2 drops under the tongue, 3–4 times a day or as required. And/or add 4–6 drops in cup of warm water, shake, and sip throughout the day.

Leucorrhoea (Vaginal Discharge)

Increased vaginal secretions are common.

HOMEOPATHY

The remedies below are for when the discharge is becoming unpleasant and potentially intolerable.

- Copious white leucorrhoea with backache: Calcarea ova-testa

- Leucorrhoea with urgent urination and abdominal-thigh pain: Mag mur
- Leucorrhoea with constipation and ruddy complexion: Natrum mur
- Milky discharge; becomes watery/acrid/burning: Pulsatilla
- Like thick slimy egg-white and green clothing stains: Bovista
- Copious clear-white and unnaturally hot: Borax
- Greenish and thick, or profuse, watery and offensive: Sepia
- Thick and corrosive: Sabina
- Yellow, offensive, acrid and causing itching/burning: Kreosotum
- Burning and yellow clothing stains: Calc carb
- Yellow-green discharge with excessive vulva itching and pelvic bearing-down sensation: Sepia
- Violently corrosive vulva itching, and very offensive yellow discharge staining clothing and lying/sitting feels better than standing: Kreosotum
- Discharge odour able to be smelt at a distance: Hepar sulph
- Postcoital burning/stinging: Staphysagria
- General combo blend: Pulsatilla, Sepia, Candida alb, Kreosotum, Hepar sulph. Take 2 drops sublingually 3–4 times a day or as required. And/or mix 4–6 drops in cup of warm water, shake, and sip throughout the day; and is okay to douche the vagina.
- Do *not* use OTC douche products (which can worsen the imbalance).

Lumbar Lordosis (Backache)

HERBALISM/NUTRITION

- Calcium phosphate supplement (many women have low calcium), and a superior magnesium supplement, and Schuessler Tissue Salt No. 8 Mag Phos (the muscle-relaxant nutrient) and Tissue Salt No. 1 Calc Fluor (the elasticity nutrient)
- Diet that reduces uric acid levels
- Visit with a chiropractor to assist neglected pelvic-movement muscles
- If back pain still not relieving, see an osteopath, masseuse and/or Bowen therapist.

HOMEOPATHY

- Main remedy: Kali carb
- With sense of weakness and dragging in the loins: Kali carb
- With difficulty walking and bruises sensation: Bellis and Arnica
- Combo blend for *Back, Ligament and Pelvic discomfort*; and for *Symphysis Pubis Dysfunction and restless legs*: Zincum met, Trillium, Calc phos, Kali carb and Aesculus hip. Take 2 drops under the tongue 3–4 times a day as required. And/or mix 4–6 drops in cup of warm water, shake, and sip throughout the day.

Nausea/Vomiting (Morning Sickness)

HERBALISM/NUTRITION

- Avoid large, heavy meals – grazing little and often is best solution – eat small frequent meals; and endeavour to eat asap after vomiting

- Nibbling on dried fruits and small protein snacks such almonds assists to maintain even blood-sugar levels
- Fats and cheese can help settle the tummy (but not to be eaten all day)
- Drinking freshly made hot cup of honey, lemon, fresh ginger and cardamom. (Honey maintains blood sugar; lemon is a natural energy boost; fresh ginger aids digestion and body toxicity; cardamon calms the stomach, circulates qi and inhibits vomiting.)
- Schuessler Tissue Salts No. 4 Ferr Phos (first-aid oxygen boost) and No. 12 Silica (cleanser and conditioner) as a natural energy boost
- Schuessler Tissue Salts Comb-S for stomach upsets, biliousness, queasiness, sick headaches and allied conditions
- Walking and getting lots of fresh air
- If unbearable, or persists into the second trimester, see herbalist or naturopath or traditional Chinese medicine therapist
- Acupuncture is also well proven to reduce the symptoms of morning sickness.
- Acupressure point P6 is found about two inches (about 5cm, or three fingers) above your crease on the palm side of your wrist, right in the middle (between the tendons). Seasickness acupressure bracelets work well.

ESSENTIAL OIL

Ginger essential oil can be a must for morning sickness. Dilute with fractionated coconut oil and apply 1–3 drops on the ears (outside only), down the jawbone and on the soles of the feet. Can be diffused into the air, or applied to the hands, and inhaling soaked tissue/cotton-wool. Plus applying a drop on the pillow before going to sleep at night.

HOMEOPATHY

There are many homeopathic remedies for morning sickness. A favourite is to combine Sepia, Natrum mur, Pulsatilla, Arsenicum alb and Capsicum. Use before getting out of bed, before cooking meals, before riding in a car, and put a couple of drops in a bottle of water, shake, and sip all day.

- At the sight and smell of food, lethargy, anger at partner: Sepia
- With early-pregnancy headaches, and dehydration from fluid imbalance: Natrum mur
- That needs fresh air, feeling faint in hot room, and worse for travelling in a car: Pulsatilla
- With fear of finances/losing a job or extreme weakness: Arsenicum alb
- With homesickness: Capsicum
- Constant, with copious saliva and unrelieved by vomiting: Ipecac
- Worse for lying down: Ipecac
- With cutting pains around the umbilicus: Ipecac
- With bearing-down sensation: Nux vomica
- From overindulgence in rich foods: Nux vomica
- With overheating: Pulsatilla
- With aversion to tight clothing at the abdomen: Nux vomica
- From arduous-feeling pregnancy: Sepia
- Better with fresh air: Pulsatilla
- Nausea unrelieved by vomiting: Ipecac
- With moist white tongue: Pulsatilla

- Food rejected as soon as taken: Ipecac or Nux vomica
- Sick feeling night and day without vomiting: Tabacum
- Incessant nausea with/without vomiting: Petroleum
- With much flatulence (assists digestive issues): Calc fluor
- If normal remedies ineffectual, then see classical homeopath to diagnose constitution.

Oedema (puffy cankles)

HERBALISM/NUTRITION

- A mineral combo supplement that provides electrolytes to assist to eliminate the fluid, plus sipping more water throughout the day
- Schuessler Tissue Salt No. 11 Nat Sulph for water elimination as a natural diuretic
- Increase protein in diet (almost to protein-only)
- Dandelion and parsley supplements
- If no improvement, see a herbalist or naturopath or masseuse.

ESSENTIAL OIL

Dilate 1–2 drops of grapefruit/cypress with tablespoon fractionated coconut oil and apply to puffy 'cankles'.

HOMEOPATHY

- Standard simple remedy: Apis
- Second option: Natrum mur

Painful Fetal Movements

Main Homeopathic remedies: Arnica (and Sepia)

Palpitations

HOMEOPATHY

If medical tests are all normal, then heart palpitations can occur through stress and/or "someone is hurting my heart" feelings, such as:

- Grief: Ignatia
- Over-sensitive: Pulsatilla
- Loss of independence: Sepia
- Dominated abusive relationship: Staphysagria
- Long-term grievances: Natrum mur
- Disappointment, grief, loss of a loved one/family/community/work: Ignatia
- Pressure from work/meeting deadlines: Nux vomica
- Male-dominance/father issues/male work colleagues/male members of the family/community: Kali carb
- Female-dominance/mother issues/female work colleagues/female members of the family/community: Kali mur

PUPPP Rash (Itchy Abdomen)

(Pruritic urticarial papules and plaques of pregnancy)

Important reminder: Nocturnal itching of the hand palms and feet soles should always be regarded as potentially serious obstetric cholestasis.

HERBALISM/NUTRITION

A high-strength omega-3 plus an inner-health "eczema relief" type product (designed to help with itching skin).

ESSENTIAL OIL

Apply topically lavender essential oil (or a therapist-created serenity blend)

HOMEOPATHY

- Main remedies: Apis, Rhus tox, Sulphur and Urtica urens
- Intense pregnancy itching: Urtica urens
- Intense allergy-itching: Apis
- Itchy legs: Rhus tox
- Nerve irritability causing scratching: Hypericum
- Combine all the above three (even also adding in Dolichos pruriens), taking 2 drops under the tongue 3–4 times a day or as required. And/or adding 4–6 drops in a cup of warm water, shake, and sip throughout the day, and apply to affected areas.
- Note: Important to keep the bowel moving regularly.

Restless Legs

Main Homeopathic remedy: Rhus tox

Rhinitis and Sinusitis (stuffy nose)

HOMEOPATHY

- Main remedies: Kali bich and Sepia
- Need to clear the air passages: Silica
- Mucus is thick with blocked ears (especially from flying): Kali mur
- Mucus is thick and green-coloured: Pulsatilla
- Mucus is thick and yellow-coloured: Sepia
- Need to fluid re-balance: Natrum mur

- Watery mucus: Hydrastis

Sciatica (leg pain from lower back)

Trauma generally caused by baby's position resulting in nerve pain radiating from lower-back down one or both legs.

HERBALISM/NUTRITION

- A superior magnesium supplement combined with Schuessler Tissue Salt No. 8 Mag Phos, which is a muscle-relaxant nutrient, and Schuessler Tissue Salt Comb-A (insomnia remedy), which is also helpful for sciatica, neuralgia, neuritis, and restless sleep from muscle-cramps or inflammations.
- Primarily sciatica does require a "mechanical" remedy, such as an osteopath, chiropractic, Bowen therapist or masseuse.

ESSENTIAL OIL

Roman chamomile, helichrysum and thyme. Dilute 5–10 drops with tablespoon fractionated coconut oil, and massage in a few drops onto the spine's lower back, buttocks, legs and feet soles.

HOMEOPATHY

- Main remedies: Cimic, Coffea, Kali bich, Kali carb and Rhus tox
- Sciatica shooting pains: Hypericum (and possibly Mag Phos also helpful)
- If nerve pain around the abdomen/groin: Bellis/Cimic
- If with general aches and pains: Arnica

- Trauma mix (e.g. Aconite, Arnica and Stramonium)
- Note: Check fetal position

SPD (Symphysis Pubis Dysfunction)

Uterine "growing" aches/pubic symphysis separation dysfunction, collectively resulting in pelvic girdle pain

HERBALISM/NUTRITION

- Check diet. Bowel gut imbalances and dehydration can aggravate (herbalist consult may assist with micronutrients).
- Additionally, a superior magnesium supplement, and Schuessler Tissue Salt No. 8 Mag Phos (muscle relaxant) can also assist.
- Temporary relief by lying on the right side with something under the hip
- Generally, the most effective cures are "mechanical" therapies such as massage, chiropractic, osteopath, and Bowen therapy may reduce symptoms
- Improved/adapted positional-mobilisation knowledge can also assist
- Acupuncture also has a solid history of reducing pregnancy pelvic-girdle pain – as do pregnancy support wraps (e.g. the Smileybelt™).

HOMEOPATHY

Homeopathy integrated with acupuncture and chiropractic care can help relieve many symptoms.

- Main remedy: Calc phos
- Combo blend for perineal muscle and ligament support:

Causticum, Gelsemium, Lilium tig and Arctium lappa. Take 2 drops under the tongue 3–4 times a day as required. And/or mix 4–6 drops in cup of warm water, shake, and sip throughout the day.

- Combo blend for back, ligament and pelvic discomfort; and for symphysis pubis dysfunction and restless legs: Zincum met, Trillium pen, Calc phos, Kali carb and Aesculus hip. Take 2 drops under the tongue 3–4 times a day as required. And/or mix 4–6 drops in cup of warm water, shake, and sip throughout the day.
- With sore/bruising from fetal movements: Bellis
- Stretched-ligament feeling with restlessness: Rhus tox
- Remedy Trillium pen is the main go-to for SPD. Also restless-legs pelvic-pain; for the pelvis/sacroiliac joints "rattling-cage, feeling-loose, falling-apart-in-two-halves" feelings that improve with tight bandaging; intense sacral backache; "gone-ness" abdominal sensation (diastasis recti).
- Remedy Aesculus hip ideal for: lower-back pain with muscle inflammation; constant monotonous backache; lumbar/sacral pain with back stiffness; tearing-pain in lower back/hips/coccyx; difficulty bending down; difficulty rising after sitting for long; and walking impossible due to excruciating pain.
- Remedy Calc phos ideal for: sore pain in the sacroiliac symphyses (caused by relaxin hormone); back sensitive to draughts; back pain when lifting/straining; visually obvious increased curvature of the spine; tearing-shooting tenderness/aches in the spine/limbs.
- Remedy Kali carb ideal for: sensation as if the back/hips/knees/legs would give way; back pain relieved by lying on a hard surface (e.g. the floor); back pain aggravated by walking/standing/sitting-upright; and hip-to-knee

pain (especially right-sided).

- Remedy Zincum met ideal for: restless legs; stiff gait with spasmodic motions; and walking flat-footed (stepping onto the full sole).
- Inability to walk in late pregnancy (due to relaxin effect on pelvic ligaments): Bellis
- Spurious (false) pains: Caul

Thrush (Vaginal)

LIFESTYLE

- Carbohydrate sugars are always implicated, so best drastically reduced.
- Swabbing topically with rice vinegar.

ESSENTIAL OILS

Melaleuca and lavender (diffuse or apply diluted to area)

HOMEOPATHY

- Main remedy: Borax
- Itchy vulva: Ambra
- Mouth washed 2–3 hourly: Borax

Urinary Tract Infections

With UTIs' ability to cause uterine irritability (potentially pre-term labour), recurrent UTIs should not be treated lightly, and are an alert for an obstetric consultation. Antibiotics strongly recommended.

HERBALISM/NUTRITION

- Garlic, of course, and few doses of zinc
- Add in "inner health"/"bladder support" type supplements
- Increase protein intake
- Recurrent UTIs – also see a naturopath/herbalist

ESSENTIAL OIL

Lemongrass and cedarwood

HOMEOPATHY (in addition to antibiotics)

- Main remedy: Cantharis
- "Honeymoon" UTI/vaginitis: Staphysagria
- With stinging and burning: Cantharis
- With incontinence from slightest exertion: Causticum

Vaginitis

Vaginal inflammation with discharge, itching and/or pain.

- For yeast infections: (e.g. Candida albicans) refer 'Thrush' section
- For Bacterial vaginosis/Trichomoniasis the main oral Homeopathic remedies are Kreosotum, Pulsatilla and Sepia

Uterine Growth (minor pains)

Main Homeopathic remedies: Arnica and Bellis

Varicose Veins

NATUROPATHY

- Schuessler Tissue Salt Comb-L (for circulatory disorders) is great for veins, piles, water retention, and impaired tissue oxygenation
- Massage with pilewort cream and/or plantain salve
- Comfrey oil is helpful to reduce pain and infection
- Issues are primarily anatomical/mechanical. With chronic issues consult with herbalist/naturopath, and masseuse.

ESSENTIAL OIL

Cypress, lemongrass and lemon. Add 3–5 drops of oils to tablespoon fractionated coconut oil, and massage above the veins towards the heart, gently applying from the ankles working up the legs. (Consistent application for an extended period is key.)

HOMEOPATHY

Homeopathy cannot cure varicose veins – it can only support unwanted symptoms and prevent inflammation.

- Main remedies: Calc fluor, Hamamelis, Pulsatilla and Sepia
- Use the haemorrhoids combo remedy and/or trauma mix (e.g. Aconite, Arnica and Stramonium)
- If veins appear lax and weak: Calc fluor

Pregnancy Pathophysiology

Important note

All the conditions below are not "normal" so require an obstetric consultation as part of their medical management. Consequentially, the following holistic treatments and remedies are generally *complementary* (not *alternative*) to modern obstetric care plans, i.e. integrative maternity health. The therapies below do *not* replace vigilant specialist obstetric management of complex complications.

Antenatal Depression

Refer *Depression & Anxiety Disorders* topic within the Postnatal section for management, treatment and remedies.

Antepartum Haemorrhage (Vaginal bleeding)

Although APHs are not uncommon, they are also never "normal", and always require obstetric consultation.

HERBALISM

Consultation with medical herbalist (cayenne pepper can be useful).

HOMEOPATHY

Consultation with classical homeopath could be beneficial. Focus can especially be on treating any levels of emotional anxiety.

Cholestasis

ICP (intrahepatic cholestasis of pregnancy)

Cholestasis is a serious medical condition diagnosed by LFT and SBA blood tests. Dietary advice, exercise, massage and acupuncture can also potentially assist. Commonest symptom: nocturnal itchy palms and soles.

HOMEOPATHY

- For intense nocturnal itching (and liver support): Dolichos pru
- Combo remedy: Urtica urens, Apis, Dolichos pru and Hypericum. Take 2 drops sublingually 3–4 times a day or as required. And/or add 4–6 drops in cup of warm water, shake, and sip throughout the day; and apply to affected areas.
- HyperCal (Hypericum-Calendula) cream to affected areas, and massage abdomen clockwise 3–4 times a day to keep bowel moving.

Food Poisoning

Main Homeopathic remedy: Arsenicum alb

Genital Herpes

Vaginal birth not recommended for active herpes.

Main Homeopathic remedies: Medorrhinum, Natrum sulph and Sepia

Gestational Diabetes Mellitus

With a GDM mother maintaining her blood sugars in the normal range by diet alone, the fetus is then fundamentally unaffected by the GDM. Any complementary support to assist her to achieve this is potentially invaluable. A naturopathic multi-disciplinary approach can be best:

NATUROPATHY

- Diet consult with nutritionist and become aware of nil-calorie, non-synthetic foods such as stevia sweetener and shirataki noodles
- Pregnancy wellness consult with medical herbalist for a customised supplement regime
- Pregnancy diabetes consult with acupuncturist

HOMEOPATHY

Constitution consult with classical homeopath for a customised tincture regime

- Main remedies: Phos and Pulsatilla
- GDM with suffering from grief: Ignatia
- GDM with history of overindulgence: Nux vomica
- For first-trimester morning sickness: see 'Nausea/ Vomiting' section earlier
- For first-trimester hyperemesis (e.g. "keeping nothing down" for 2–3 days): a general medical consult is warranted for IV fluids rehydration and anti-emetic medication prescription
- For second-trimester hyperemesis: an obstetric specialist consult is always warranted.

ACUPUNCTURE

Acupuncture can oftentimes be of great assistance in reducing symptoms and enhancing the quality of the woman's pregnancy journey enjoyment.

HOMEOPATHY

- Main remedy: Ipecac
- General blend remedy: Asafoetida, Gossypium, Natrum mur and Ferrum phos. Take 2 drops sublingually 3–4 times a day or as required. And/or add 4–6 drops to cup warm water, shake, and sip throughout the day.
- Good all-round remedy for desperate cases of vomiting continuously, severe nausea, violent retching, and smell/thought of food intolerable: Symphoricarpus rac.
- Note: Constitution consult with classical homeopath likely also needed.

IUGR (Intrauterine Growth Restriction)

Physiological SGA (small for gestational age) fetuses tend to have a sub-optimum maternal lifestyle (e.g. smoker, work high-stress factors, diet, lifestyle). To assist to prevent the SGA becoming an IUGR, a naturopathic care plan can be beneficial, along with the homeopathic remedy Calc phos.

IUGR fetuses can be pathologically complicated. Thus, full diagnosis with complex ultrasound scans (including placental dopplers and liquor levels) and a customized growth chart are critical.

With the specialist obstetric medical consult prognosis, then complementary therapists can create a customized support plan.

HOMEOPATHY

Calc phos is a popular remedy to improve general fetal failure to grow.

Malpresentation/Malposition

35+ weeks gestation, and lie is breech, transverse, oblique or unstable.

ACUPUNCTURE

Moxibustion in particular can assist obstetric manipulation management.

ESSENTIAL OIL

Myrrh is associated with improving fetal lie (topically and aromatically).

HOMEOPATHIC BREECH REMEDIES UP TO 37 WEEKS

- Main malposition remedy: Pulsatilla
- One dose Pulsatilla 3 times a day, repeat after 48 hours, then repeat every 3–5 days until baby turns
- Stop if large movement felt
- Do not combine with acupuncture or moxibustion.

HOMEOPATHIC TURNING A BREECH REMEDY FROM 37 WEEKS

Combo blend of Pulsatilla, Tuberc koch, Borax and Natrum mur.

- Instruct woman to lie down in a restful place, and put her hands onto her abdomen to "connect" with her baby's movements

- Take 2 drops sublingually and repeat 3–4 times (every 15 minutes)
- Woman may feel slight movement
- If woman feels larger movement and suspects her baby has turned, she should go for a walk, taking a homeopathic birth mix with her
- If baby has not turned, woman can repeat this process every evening
- Avoid refined foods, carbohydrates, and fruit (especially oranges and strawberries).

HOMEOPATHY SUPPORTING AN ECV (external cephalic version)

- Use a birth mix (see Intrapartum section as an example)
- Initial dose: 2 drops sublingually prior to procedure
- Repeat dose if baby is not turning easily
- Repeat dose once baby successfully cephalic
- Repeat dose daily until birth, with a daily 20-minute powerwalk

OTHER HOMEOPATHIC MALPOSITION REMEDIES

- Breech with oligohydramnios/polyhydramnios: Natrum mur
- Breech unstable lie: Tuberc koch
- Breech and no engagement: Borax/Gelsemium
- Breech (to change the shape of the uterus): Pulsatilla
- Fetal fear of descent: Boron/Gelsemium
- Unstable lie: Tuberc koch
- Transverse lie: Arnica (also lifestyle, e.g. desk worker, driver)

Oligohydramnios/Polyhydramnios

OLIGOHYDRAMNIOS:

Abnormally decreased waters around fetus. Commonest causes: placental insufficiency, fetal abnormality, or premature rupture of membranes (waters breaking pre-term).

POLYHYDRAMNIOS:

- Abnormally increased waters around fetus. Commonest causes: maternal gestational diabetes, or fetal disease
- A multi-discipline approach recommended, including the basics of seeing a medical herbalist, acupuncturist, and classical homeopath
- Homeopathy for Oligohydramnios/polyhydramnios homeopathy: Natrum mur
- Diet for Polyhydramnios: reduce dietary carbohydrates

PET (Pre-eclampsic Toxaemia)

Hypertension with other dysfunction (e.g. proteinuria, low platelets, and/or abnormal renal/liver function).

As well as obstetric medical care, a multi-discipline approach is *strongly* recommended, including the basics of seeing a medical herbalist, acupuncturist, and classical homeopath – as well as dietary advice, meditation and gentle yoga.

NATUROPATHY

- Herbalism: consultation with qualified medical herbalist can potentially be of significant benefit (such as traditional Chinese medicine)

- Lifestyle: dietary advice, meditation, yoga and acupuncture can also all potentially greatly assist.

HOMEOPATHY

- Main remedies: Apis, Colchicum, Nux vomica and Sulphur
- Blood-pressure white-coat syndrome: Natrum mur
- With impatient personality: Nux vomica/Sepia
- Proteinuria without hypertension: increase diet protein and homeopathic tincture Sulphur
- Consultation with classical homeopath as support to bring constitution back to homeostatic equilibrium.

LIFESTYLE

Doing as little stress-related activities (mental, physical or emotional) including housework and going to work ... time to simply "make a dent on the couch".

Phlebitis (Vein inflammation)

Obstetric consultation essential.

Main Homeopathic remedies: Belladonna, Bryonia, Carb veg, Hamamelis and Pulsatilla

PICA Disorder (Compulsion to eat non-food items)

Main Homeopathic remedy: Calc carb

PIH (Pregnancy-induced Hypertension)

As soon as borderline/confirmed hypertension is diagnosed, a holistic multi-discipline approach is recommended, including particularly seeing a medical herbalist, acupuncturist, and classical homeopath – as well as dietary advice, meditation and gentle yoga. Doing so can potentially be of significant benefit to stabilize/reverse the diagnosis, and improve prognosis by possibly completely preventing pre-eclampsia/eclampsia.

ESSENTIAL OIL

Cypress diluted 1:1 with fractionated coconut oil, and 2 drops applied to the feet soles and abdomen daily. Also, diffusing cypress oil (or inhaling it directly from the bottle).

HOMEOPATHY

- Common general remedy: Natrum mur, 3 times a day
- Potentially alternating with: Apis.

Placenta Previa/Low-lying Placenta/Vasa Previa

Formally from 32 weeks, when the placenta extends wholly or partly into the womb lower-segment, this requires obstetric management including defining it as a major or minor placenta previa (i.e. over the os or just low-lying) and whether it penetrates through the uterine decidua basalis/myometrium (i.e. accreta, increta, percreta).

However, assistance from complementary therapies (particularly acupuncture and homeopathy) should begin as soon a potential placental issue is reported (i.e. typically after the anatomy scan).

Acupuncture is generally quite successful, especially in minor cases of previa.

Homeopathy has many different potential remedies for a low-lying placenta, which require a consultation for the correct constitutional fit (oftentimes prescribing Nux vomica).

Post-dates (Prolonged Pregnancy 41½–42 Weeks)

In general terms, ideally a healthy normal pregnancy is referred for an obstetric consultation at around 41½ weeks, to be booked for an induction at 42 weeks. (See 'Labour and Birth Preparation' section.)

A multi-disciplinary approach can potentially greatly assist, particularly herbalism, homeopathy and acupuncture. The below are specific examples to potentially assist the body to commence spontaneous labour.

HERBALISM

Nature's Sunshine "5-W" herbal capsules, and evening primrose oil (orally and vaginally) can together assist tremendously, as can seeing a medical herbalist.

HOMEOPATHY

From 40 weeks onwards a daily 60-minute regimen of alternating remedies Caul and Cimic every 10 minutes (i.e. 3 doses of each over one hour).

Note: Do *not* use Caul once contractions start.

Recurrent Miscarriage

Women with a history of recurrent miscarriages, as well as potentially being under specialist obstetric/gynaecological infertility care, are recommended to *also* be under the care of a maternity-specializing medical herbalist (e.g. Western, traditional Chinese medicine or Indian Ayurvedic) and acupuncturist, for enhanced fertility health and wellness. Additional therapies:

ESSENTIAL OIL

The oils of frankincense, grapefruit and geranium (massaged and added to bathwater) are associated with maintaining pregnancies.

HOMEOPATHY

- First-trimester miscarriage-prevention: consultation to assess constitution (commonly poor diet creating insulin resistance)
- Second-trimester miscarriage-prevention remedy: Sepia

SGA (Small for Gestational Age)

See IUGR in this chapter.

Stretch Mark Prevention

Stretch marks appear in 90 percent of pregnancies because there is no single magical panacea for preventing them. The severity is mostly genetically influenced (whether the woman's mother and grandmothers had them). Treating from the inside out, the combination of protein-rich diet with a good daily multi-vitamin multi-mineral is beneficial. Treating from the outside in, moisturising belly-oil and belly-butter products such as BioOil®.

For women with a strong family history of stretch marks: Homeopathic oral remedy: Calc fluor.

Threatened Pre-term Labour

This topic crosses over into the Intrapartum section. However, two excellent homeopathic remedies include:

- TPTL after a shock or fright: Aconite
- TPTL after a fall with twisting/straining: Rhus tox.

Labour and Birth Preparation

Cascade of Intervention vs Cascade of Normalcy

Midwives prescribing, and expectant women using, labour *partus preparatus* herbs is as ancient as birth itself ... but somehow in the West, that exquisitely timeless and eternal role of the midwife has predominantly morphed (through protocols, procedures and political correctness) into most of today's midwives being more skilled in medicalized induction than naturopathic induction; and more educated on the modern management of obstetric complexities than educated on the traditional prevention of pregnancy complications.

Midwifery of course *had* to go down the rabbit hole of empirical medical education, but surely not at the almost complete cost of losing respect for its own historical, time-honoured herbalism knowledge ... but unfortunately, it is blatantly apparent much of our collective, over the past century, forgot to leave ourselves a path of crumbs showing the way to return to being truly "wholistic" in our therapeutic modality wisdom.

The fact remains, Gaia (Mother Earth) provides an *enormous amount of safer options* for our clients, that lie in-between the two divergent poles of:

Using nothing

vs

ARM → epidural → IV oxytocin and continuous CTG

A critical part of our role as birth facilitators providing informed consent is to ensure our clients are aware of *all* their options, so they can avoid the almost unbridled, and oftentimes potentially preventable, obstetric interventions. These are the most common consequences of inductions, augmentations and epidurals.

- Failure to progress (not fully dilatating, often due to lack of the gravity-assisting maternal leaning-forward positions normal to natural labour, plus relying on synthetically induced contractions).
- Obstructed labour (a mal-flexed baby's head failing to descend, often due to hours of the mother lying semi-recumbent on her back with epidural and continuous CTG cardiotocography).
- Fetal distress (the "tired" baby, consequential to the longer pharmaceutically augmented labours – in drastic contrast to the shorter length of natural spontaneous labours after use of *partus preparatus*, or birth-preparation, naturopathy).

This is the routine widespread *Cascade of Intervention* that is far from a natural, normal labour.

- Artificial rupture of membranes (ARM) →
- Site the Epidural →
- Commence the Oxytocin drip and commence continuous CTG/fetal heartrate monitoring (because the interventions have medically altered the labour from *low-risk* to *high-risk*).

Common outcomes from above interventions: trial of instrumental vaginal delivery, otherwise on to:

- "Failure to progress" (cervix failing to dilatate) → C-section surgical delivery
- Or "Fetal distress" (baby tired of long labour) → C-section
- Or "Obstructed labour" (baby failing to descend) → C-section.

With, for example, the common 35–40 per cent C-section rates in Western hospitals, that logically equates to at least a 50 per cent rate amongst primips (first births). Then add in the forcep and ventouse instrumental deliveries, and for most first-time mothers-to-be, they can end up having about a two-thirds chance of their baby experiencing a dramatic emergency obstetric delivery as their traumatic arrival into this world. And people ... that is *nuts*! **Every instrumental and surgical delivery is an event of *trauma* for the baby (and their mother).**

When you routinely work in the primary care birthing setting seeing healthy, normal women experiencing beautiful natural births, trust me that you will also routinely witness newborns who don't cry – instead they just look around the room with big blinks, almost smiling ... I swear for many of them, if they could purr, they would. Then, within minutes they self-latch beautifully onto their mother's breast. (And when women experience a positive childbirth, and their baby thrives, it is *extremely rare* for those women to later suffer from postnatal depression.)

Whether we are an obstetrician, midwife, doula or childbirth educator, our *job* is to ensure our clients are empowered to understand *what they can proactively do* to enhance the *Cascade of Normalcy* for their baby's birth experience ... to "line up all their ducks in a row".

And this all begins way, *way* before the first contraction!

IIMHCO's 7 Gold Standards to Best-practice Birth Preparation

(International Integrative Maternity HealthCare Org)

1. Your client receives childbirth education beyond the routine prenatal course ("average" education = "average" outcomes). Such as having the MothersWise Organic Birth.

2. Your client proactively learns about her natural pain-relief options, such as hydrotherapy for labour; the extraordinarily effective natural pain-management technique termed hypnobirthing (i.e. meditative labour); and prenatal optimal fetal positioning techniques.

3. Your client reads great literature on natural childbirth, e.g. *Ina May's Guide to Childbirth* by Ina May Gaskin, *New Active Birth* by Janet Balaskas, and the childbirth chapter of Kathy Fray's *Oh Baby ... Birth, Babies & Motherhood Uncensored*.

4. Your client is fully empowered with familiarity of the physiological *three stages of childbirth* (labour, birth, after-birth), and the *three phases of labour* (latent, active, transition).

5. Your client's "birth-support crew" are also fully familiarized with the same information: especially knowing fear produces adrenaline (the "enemy" of labour's oxytocin) ... and the more anxiety in the birthing room (be it the mother or her support people) then the slower her dilatation, and the subsequent increased

need for epidural anaesthesia.

6. Your client has received full "informed consent" prenatal education on the negative obstetric consequences of opting for an epidural during low-risk spontaneous natural contractions, and how it changes the labour from obstetrically low-risk to obstetrically high-risk, resulting in increased chances of a lengthened labour, and fetal distress, and failure-to-progress, and obstructed labour, and instrumental forceps/ventouse delivery, and/or surgical Caesarean section.

7. Your client is aware of the prenatal naturopathic herbal therapies, homeopathic remedies, and GLA EPO oils available, that can effectively "tone" her uterus and "ripen" her cervix, to assist her body to spontaneously go into labour at term, with effective contractions and efficient dilatation.

The Three Third-trimester Birth-preparation "Musts"

These birth-prep "musts" gently support healthy women with normal pregnancies to birth naturally.

No. 1: Pre-birth Naturopathy

Wherever you are in the world, it is important to seek out the local producer of herbal *partus preparatus* supplements.

A personal all-time favourite combo is Nature's Sunshine "5-W" (5-W stands for last five weeks of the pregnancy). This is a well-loved traditional herbal tonic blend of square vine, dong quai, butcher's broom, black cohosh and red raspberry; taken from the 35th week of pregnancy until labour.

Rather than following the packaging's simplified instructions of 2 capsules 3 times a day from 35 weeks onwards, I recommend an even gentler increase of:

- 35–37 weeks: 1 capsule 3 times a day
- 37–40 weeks: 2 capsules 3 times a day
- From 40 weeks: 3 capsules 4 times a day

Because the date of spontaneous labour is unpredictable, then at the time of giving birth the woman will usually have some leftover 5-W capsules. These will not to be wasted. She simply continues to consume them until they have run out, which will assist uterine involution.

Note: If it is being suggested by the obstetrician that an induction of labour prior to 42 weeks is medically indicated, then our recommendation is the woman taking the full dose on the packaging.

No. 2: Pre-birth Homeopathy

Again, wherever you are in the world, it is important to seek out the local producer of homeopathy tinctures, to get access to at least a birth prep mix.

One of my personal favorites is NaturoPharm's "Pre-Birth" blend that includes Caul (Caulophyllum), Cimic, Arnica, Pulsatilla and Gelsemium, and is used from 37 weeks onwards for general wellbeing and to reduce false labour.

NaturoPharm also produces a "Birth-Aid" blend, which

should be used as soon as labour contractions begin, then throughout the labour, and for the first two to three days following birth. It is a combo of Arnica, Bellis, Hypericum and Hamamelis. I have found this remedy *especially* useful for exhausted primips in the second stage, when contractions begin to wane in length, strength or frequency – *hey presto*, her body and mind are boosted, and *voila*, the baby is born.

Global British-Kiwi midwife Irene Chain-Kalinowski is an extremely senior homeopathic midwife, who alongside obstetrician homeopathic guru colleagues has created a customized *My Body My Baby* birth-mix blend consisting of Caul, Cimic, Pulsatilla and Gelsemium. Again, it tones the uterus, supports cervical ripening, assists fetal positioning, and helps the mother to cope with the discomforts of her baby descending into her pelvis.

Dosage:

- 36–40 weeks: 2 drops sublingually combined with a 20-minute powerwalk
- Over 40 weeks: 2 drops sublingually twice daily (before the powerwalk, and before going to bed).

Additional homeopathic remedies useful from 36 weeks are:

- Woman nervous about pending childbirth: Act rac
- Woman fearful about pending childbirth: Gelsemium.

No. 3: Evening Primrose GLA Oil (Gamma-linolenic Acid)

And finally, high-strength EPO (Evening Primrose Oil) capsules, which are a natural source of the omega-6 fatty-acid GLA, the levels of which we recommend boosting from 37 weeks onwards, again to help tone the womb, ripen the cervix, initiate term labour, and promote easier birth.

Derived from the evening primrose seeds, the oil is usually sold in capsule form and contains gamma-linolenic acid, which gently assists the body to naturally produce its own prostaglandins to soften the cervix.

Interesting aside: A large percentage of the general population are unable to effectively produce their own optimum levels of GLA, most commonly due to dietary deficiencies, alcohol abuse, smoking, viral infections, and/or medical conditions. Adding GLA into the diet can also improve production of long-chain omega-6 essential fatty acids. These omega-3 and omega-6 EFAs are metabolized by the body into hormones called eicosanoids (i.e. prostaglandin is an eicosanoid). Hypothesis: Is this perhaps why some women fail to go into spontaneous labour?

Some birth practitioners advocate EPO oral-only use is fully effective. Other birth practitioners advocate topical *per vaginal* use too. Personally, I believe *both* have a positive influence. (Each birth practitioner formulates their own practice style.) But either way, it has been strongly concluded women who use EPO have a softer, supple, more stretchable cervix (and anecdotally there may also be some health benefits to prevent cervical oedema).

Oral dose recommendations of the 1000 mg capsules vary from practitioner to practitioner, but as a generally accepted summary:

- At 36-37 weeks: 1 capsule at night
- At 37-38 weeks: 2 capsules at night

- At 38-40 weeks: 2 capsules twice daily
- At 40+ weeks: 2 capsules 3 times daily

For women opting to also use EPO topically *per vagina* (especially for women who know the obstetric medical system may not give their body until its full 42 weeks' gestation to spontaneously go into natural labour), the general dose is one capsule gently inserted to the top of the vagina each evening at bedtime. The woman punctures a hole in the capsule before inserting, and typically the capsule falls out in the morning when she goes to the toilet.

Note: Like "5-W", any leftover EPO capsules at the time of birth will not be wasted. The woman can continue to use them up over the postpartum period for enhanced recovery and wellbeing.

For women with medical complexities or obstetric complications

These women can still potentially take advantage of herbalism, homeopathy and evening primrose oil – in fact, one could say they are in even greater need of such extra support – however it is strongly recommended they obtain a customized care-plan prepared by a professionally qualified naturopathic herbalist and classical homeopath. As well as strongly considering to regularly see an acupuncturist.

Pizzas are delivered. Strong women give birth.

Joan Donley, leading NZ midwife

The Intrapartum (Childbirth)

'Wholistic' Preparation is the Key

BODY

It can be very beneficial for a woman to have a private consultation with a herbalist in the weeks prior to commencing labour, as they will usually provide her with a personalized array of remedies to use at various parts of her latent labour, to assist her womb to be effectively productive and her cervical dilatation not to be prolongingly protracted.

MIND AND EMOTIONS

Best practice is the woman having access to an individually created homeopathic birth blend customized to her unique constitution. However, her having access to *any* practitioner-created homeopathic birth blend mix is far, far better than having no access to any at all ... so over-the-counter birth blend homeopathic tinctures are absolutely fine.

SPIRIT

Of potentially extraordinary benefit can be the woman seeing an acupuncturist leading up to the labour, as well as her birth support person learning acupressure points (particularly reflexology, which can provide amazing pain-management relief).

HYPNOBIRTHING

Without any doubt, consistently *the* most extraordinarily powerful and mesmerizing pain-management tool I have *ever* witnessed is *hypnobirthing*.

Women have been using meditation during their labours since we have been giving birth – it is nothing new. But when a primip is deeply centred within the spellbinding "trance" of her contraction waves, I have to comment as her midwife, it is always mesmerizing how gobsmackingly quick her cervix will dilatate.

Personally, in my practice, my primips average 3–4-hour active labours, and my multips 1–2-hour active labours. This was not because of anything ground-breaking I did for them. It is always because of what the woman does for herself – particularly the magical combo of *partus preparatus* medical herbalism *and hypnobirthing meditative labour.*

Author Comment

If someone is a *Hypnobirth educator*, that does not make them a trained *Hypnotherapist*. They are simply trained in one particular method (e.g. Mongan/Lamaze) of one modality of hypnotherapy (i.e. hypnobirth). A *hypnobirther* is unable to do what a board-certified *hypnotherapist* can help with, such as issues like depression, anxiety, self-esteem, body image, etc.

The Five "Birth-rite Kit" Must-haves

Whether the labour is naturally spontaneous or medically induced; whether the woman is a primip or grand multip; whether the pregnancy is a singleton or triplets; the woman still needs to go through Labour's three phases of latent, active and transition, and Childbirth's three stages of labour, birth and after-birth – and there are very specific and amazingly supportive "must" items she should have as part of her own "Birth-rite Kit", to help her body and mind do what is needed to dilatate her cervix effectively; and birth her baby and placenta successfully; and involute her womb efficiently. And her birth practitioner teaching her this information can be prophylactically *life transformative* to both herself and her unborn baby ... it can change outcomes!

As midwives, obstetricians, doulas and childbirth educators, we are practically the biggest influencer on the rest of that woman's life as a mother, due to how exceedingly powerful the lifelong impact can be on her knowing she gave her baby a textbook-beautiful, non-traumatic birth versus knowing she gave her baby a textbook-nightmare, traumatic delivery. *We are like the publisher's editors helping her to write her life story.*

No. 1: Homeopathic Labour-birth Blend

There are various homeopathic birth-aid blends available, typically with ingredient mixes along the lines of: Arnica,

Bellis, Hypericum, Hamamelis, Gelsemium, Pulsatilla, Caul and/or Cimic.

The blends are always about giving the woman an edge to labour gently but productively, and birth gently but powerfully. (Homeopathy does not take over as pharmaceutical drugs do – it only ever enhances the body and mind to optimally do what it is inherently capable of doing.)

Generally during labour and birth, only use a homeopathic tincture every 10–20 minutes *until you see the desired signs of improvement*. After 30–40 minutes if there is no change, consider a different remedy.

Homeopathic emotional remedies and Bach's Rescue Remedy can also be very helpful for not just the woman in labour, but also her birth support people too!

UTERINE FATIGUE

As a 24/7 on-call self-employed midwife, around 40 per cent of my clients' births occurred at home or at a primary-care birth-centre facility (just over half were at the local secondary-care hospital facility). And I cannot begin to add up the hundreds of times seeing a primip who is well hydrated, but exhausted and fully dilatated, with her second-stage contractions beginning to peter off. Then within 5–15 minutes of administering a few drops of homeopathy, her contractions vividly amp up again and her spirit is radically re-energized again, and *voila*, the baby is born. I am awestruck every single time!

I cannot fathom how many *hundreds* of these women – just with a few drops of homeopathic tincture – avoided transferring to the hospital for obstetric's standard remedy of "in goes the epidural; on goes the CTG; and up goes the Synto" ... which nearly always ends up as an instrumental or surgical delivery.

No. 2: Bach's Flower "Rescue Remedy"

Rescue Remedy is a special blend of Bach's flower extracts including Rock Rose, Impatiens, Clematis, Star of Bethlehem and Cherry Plum, which together have a "near magical" ability to help balance emotions (reducing fear and anxiety).

We recommend the woman's birth-support partner adds a few drops to her drinking water during the entire labour, to help maintain a positive mood through this emotionally demanding time ... it's also marvellous for anxious birth support people too.

No. 3: Electrolyte Rehydration

Staying well hydrated (with a good electrolyte balance) is *vital* during labour for efficient cervical dilatation, effective pushing descent, and fetal wellbeing, so we recommend natural electrolyte powder drink-sachets to replace essential electrolytes lost during the "marathon" of childbirth – particularly boosting her magnesium, sodium, calcium and potassium.

Note: Sports rehydration drinks can also be effective – however even with providing very specific explanations on the difference between *sports drinks* and *energy drinks*, the wrong thing can end up packed into the woman's bag by herself or her partner – which is why getting the powder-sachets instead can be more consistently reliable.

No. 4: Lavender Essential Oil

If the woman has her own access to an array of pure essential oils, that is potentially fantastic. But if she can afford only one, then it is lavender with its calming soothing qualities ... being aromatically diffused, or a few drops on her pillows, or a few drops in the birth-pool water during labour, or sprayed as a facial-spritz, this oil is good for the soul, creating a feeling of embraced comfort.

No. 5: Music

Music can potently enable a woman to chill out (and oftentimes zone out) during her labour dilatation, assisting her to "find her centre" where contractions wash over her (instead of take over her). However, the music doesn't need to be a whale-singing, wave-breaking, bird-tweeting, waterfall-splashing cacophony of Mother Nature. In fact, in my experience, simply hours of easy-listening "normal" music helps her *normalize* her experience.

Note: You are welcome to use my Spotify "Childbirth" 200-song playlist under profile "Mark Kathy Fray". (FYI, I believe it is the unpredictable eclectic-ness of this mix of tunes that can be freeing for a woman in labour, because it is not a playlist she created filled with her specific expectations.)

First Stage: Labour Latent Phase (Early Labour)

With a long latent phase there are so many gentle options instead of the harsh use of performing an ARM breaking the waters, or commencing an oxytocin drip. Sometimes all that is needed is IV fluids, a vigorous stretch and sweep, and a few drops of the perfect homeopathic tincture, then *hey presto*, it's all on!

PROLONGED LATENT PHASE

With a rigid cx (cervix) and a woman physically sapped and emotionally depleted from a prolonged latent phase (i.e. especially with obstetric Inductions), it is always worth considering an opioid (e.g. pethidine, morphine) to allow the client a break from her unproductive contraction pain, to recover her strength. However, in my experience, a rigid cervix after latent labour rarely tends to happen with women who have invested in *Partus preparatus* (prenatal birth-prep naturopathy).

HOMEOPATHY

- *Give Arnica routinely 4–6 hourly (for stamina)*
- Cx rigid or hard: Sepia, Caul/Cham/Gelsemium
- Cx rigid and contractions weak: Caul
- Cx rigid, contractions ineffectual and woman nervous/ prostrated: Gelsemium
- Cx rigid and closed, and contractions 'intolerable': Cham

- Cx rigid, and woman restless and hot: Aconite
- Cx remaining closed despite regular contractions: Natrum mur/Staph/Cimic
- Cx not opening, despite feeling of downward pressure: Nux vomica
- Cx dilatation slow and irregular: Caul/Cimic
- Cx swollen and tight: Apis
- Cx open but contractions fading: Gelsemium/Staph/Sepia
- Contractions absent/weak (atonic uterus): Secale
- Contractions weak: Caul/Cimic/Gelsemium/Natrum mur
- Contractions weak and woman's mindset negative: China
- Contractions weak and feeble (woman "closed" on all levels): Natrum mur
- Contractions irregular, short and weak: Caul
- Contractions irregular and uncoordinated: Belladonna/Caul/Cimic
- Contractions irregular and uncoordinated from exhaustion/weakness: Secale
- Contractions slowing/stopping: Caul/Cimic/Gelsemium/Natrum mur
- Contractions changeable (irregular, weak, uncoordinated): Pulsatilla
- Labour appears to be progressing well, but cx surprisingly closed/barely open: Staphysagria

First Stage: Labour Active Phase (including Advanced-active Transitional Phase)

Obstetrically "prolonged" active labour is regarded as dilatating less than 2 cm every 4 hours for a nullipara (and half that time for a multipara). However, these protocols are based to allow for epidural-oxytocin augmented labours.

PROLONGED ACTIVE PHASE

In my substantial experience of spontaneous natural labours with women who have had proactive prenatal use of birth *partus preparatus* naturopathy, combined with a non-epidural labour supported by the birth support aids explained in this chapter plus *active mobilization*; then the outcome is *very few* women experiencing prolonged active labours. In fact, during my years as a 24/7 on-call case-loading midwife, I can count on one hand the truly prolonged active labours retrospectively caused by the rare but genuine CPD (cephalopelvic disproportion) of baby's head too large for the mother's pelvis (which I have witnessed as generally being a mixed-race baby – such as from a petite Asian woman and a large Polynesian partner).

HOMEOPATHY

- *For stamina give Arnica 4–6 hourly (or 1–2 hourly if woman needs a "second wind").*
- Vaginal examinations unusually painful: Cimic/Cham
- Contractions long, slow and painful: Arnica

- Contractions too fast and violent: Aconite/Belladonna
- Contraction pain extends to thighs: Caul/Cimic
- Contraction pain moves from side to side: Cimic
- Contraction pain cramping-shooting feeling: Mag phos/ Nux vomica
- Contraction pain sharp and "shooting up" from cx: Cimic/Sepia
- Contraction pain finishes at the throat with choking sensation: Gelsemium
- Suspected uterine exhaustion: Chloral hy
- Rim of cx left: Arnica/Bellis
- Posterior-lie premature urge to push (mild sensations): Nux vomica
- Irresistible urge to push before fully dilatated: Secale/ Nux vomica
- Deep fear stalling labour: Cimic
- Visibly entering into the transition phase of advanced-active labour: give Arnica for stamina and to provide a "second wind".
- Hypertonic (excessive) contractions: Calc phos, Caul and Mag phos
- Main 'Failure to Progress' remedies: Caul, Gelsemium and Pulsatilla

Second Stage: Birth (Pushing)

Period from fully dilatated with an irresistible urge to push, until baby born. Note: Obstetrically a "prolonged" second stage is regarded as more than 2 hours of active pushing with *no progress* for a nullipara (and half that time for a multipara).

PROLONGED SECOND STAGE

The "no progress" definition can tend to get incorrectly pigeon-holed in the hospital setting – i.e. the protocol does *not* say "baby born" within 1–2 hours, it says "no progress" in that time. In reality, with natural primip childbirth, so long as the mother is coping, and the baby is showing no signs of stress, and descent *is* occurring, it is not extraordinary for a natural second stage to take longer than 2 hours.

HOMEOPATHY

- *For stamina and a "second wind", give Arnica 1–2 hourly.*
- In need of another "second wind": Secale
- Contractions appear to be ascending baby, instead of descending: Gelsemium/Nux vomica
- Everything feeling too loose and flabby, need help to bring baby down: Secale
- "Hour-glass"contractions (strong-weak-strong): Cham/Secale/Sepia
- Contractions lacking pushing power: Pulsatilla/Cimic/Sepia
- Violent bearing-down (feeling like everything will "fall out"): Sepia

CROWNING

Of extreme assistance during crowning can be a flannel soaked in warm water with diluted drops of Calendula, applied to the stretching perineum (optionally Calendula cream also generously applied topically).

And/or Helichrysum pure essential oil applied to the perineum, prior and during crowning (e.g. diluted on the warm, wet face-cloth), can also assist to lessen tearing and bruising.

Third Stage: After-birth (Delivery of Placenta and Membranes, Plus Control of Bleeding)

NORMAL CARES

- Prophylactic prevention of RPOC given routinely immediately after baby born: Secale
- History of RPOC: prophylactic use during third stage: Arnica/Bellis/Calc fluor
- Intense nausea: Ipecac
- No contractions (atonic uterus): Caul/Cimic/Secale/ Pulsatilla
- Inadequate contractions to expel: Pulsatilla/Ipecac/ Secale
- Hysterical with each contraction: Secale
- Fruitless urges to bear down: Secale/Sepia/Nux vom
- Bleeding during third stage: Ipecac/Pulsatilla/Secale/ Belladonna
- ?RPOC feeble contractions: Secale
- ?RPOC from ?exhaustion: Arnica and Caul
- Essential oil: few drops of diluted basil oil massage on lower abdomen and feet soles
- Homeopathic "exhaustion" blend of Fluoric acid, Phos acid, Kali phos and China. Can give a sudden extra burst of natural energy to help see the woman through to delivering the placenta (2 drops sublingually during labour-birth when feeling exhausted).

Other General Support of Natural Labour and Normal Birth

Allergic Rash from Drugs/Products

Homeopathic remedy: Rhus tox

(*See also* Hypersensitivity in the next section.)

Anxious Emotions

Obviously, some level of anxious excitement is a normal emotion during the childbirth experience. However, there are times when the intensity of such feelings can leave the woman feeling emotionally debilitated, with her confidence incapacitated, and her subsequent high levels of adrenaline consequently hampering her body's oxytocin, so her mindset directly encumbering her dilatation.

This is where homeopathy in particular can have the unique ability to gently but powerfully impact the woman's emotions positively by "taking the intense edge off". This overall improvement to her self-empowerment and mental wellbeing can enable an oxytocin-dominant labour to dilatate her cervix efficiently and potentially shorten the length of her labour, thus reducing her need for obstetric interventions (and its risks of fetal distress). This then directly improves the likelihood of her and her baby experiencing a *normal, unassisted, non-traumatic birth*. It can sound cliché, but I have witnessed it hundreds and hundreds of times. *Adrenaline is the enemy of labour's oxytocin.*

The immense positive impact and lifelong benefits of

proactively supporting a labouring woman to "keep her head in a good space" and successfully continue along the natural "Cascade of Normalcy" cannot be over-emphasized!

NATUROPATHY

- Essential oils: lavender, ylang ylang, melissa, cedarwood, blue tansy, magnolia, green mandarin, yarrow can bring a sense of calm.
- Bach's flower Rescue Remedy

HOMEOPATHY

- Obvious fear and/or shock: Aconite
- Aggressive anxiety with thirst: Arsenicum alb
- Aggressive or abusive: Bell/Sepia
- Aggressive *and* abusive: Cham
- Angry and Aggressive: Cham, Nux vomica and Staphysagria
- Angry: Cham, Nux vomica/Staphysagria/Sepia
- Closed off: Natrum mur
- Despair: Sepia/Gelsemium/Cimic
- Feeling humiliated: Staphysagria/Natrum mur
- Hysterical: Gelsemium/Cimic/Pulsatilla/Sepia/ Belladonna/Ignatia
- Indifferent: Gelsemium/China/Sepia/Natrum mur
- Irritable: Apis/Cham/Nux vomica/Rhus tox/Sepia
- Wanting sympathy: Pulsatilla
- Rejecting sympathy: Sepia/Arnica
- Restless: Arsenicum alb/Acon/Rhus tox
- Restless and intense: Arsenicum alb
- Weepy: Pulsatilla/Sepia
- Says she's okay when clearly she isn't: Arnica
- Supersensitive: Belladonna

- Flushed face, dilated pupils, hot, dry: Belladonna
- Intense primitive instincts: Belladonna
- Violent reaction: Belladonna
- Craves lemonade: Belladonna
- Needy and Tearful: Pulsatilla
- Tearful and trembling: Caul
- Demands epidural/Caesarean: Cham
- Refuses examinations: Cham
- Hot, sweaty, and thirsty for cold drinks: Cham
- Sensitive to light touch and opposed to light touch: China
- Deeply fearful, 'resisting' contractions: Cimic
- Anticipatory anxiety (fear to "perform" in front of others): Gelsemium
- Weakness, trembling: Gelsemium
- Woman prefers to be left alone, intolerant of chit-chat: Natrum mur
- Acutely sensitive to humiliation: Natrum mur
- Critical and supersensitive to light/noise/smells: Nux vomica
- Mother soft and yielding in nature (weepy, clingy, apologizing, needing support): Pulsatilla
- Short mood swings of irritating and demanding: Pulsatilla
- Irritable, weepy, angry, shudders with pain, and wants to be covered: Sepia
- Belligerent behaviour and whose pregnancy featured haemorrhoids/varicose veins/incontinence: Sepia
- Sweet and compliant woman with suppressed anger: Staphysagria
- Anger/resentment to "intrusive" internal exams/procedures: Staphysagria
- Supersensitivity amplifies into humiliation/criticism:

Staphysagria

Asthma (mild)

Normal prescribed medicine and homeopathic Aconite

Chills and Tremors

Main Homeopathic remedies: Caul, Cimic, Gelsemium and Pulsatilla

Constipation

- If causing the woman grief: homeopathic Verat alb
- If hindering fetal descent, discuss consent for a quick enema or manual extraction (or simply strategic digital pressure to posterior vaginal wall may assist)

Contraction Pain Management

Also refer the labour stage in this section.

HOMEOPATHY

- Stitch-like contraction pains: Kali carb
- Centre lower-abdomen pain that moves side to side: Cimic
- Cramping-shooting contraction pains: Mag phos
- Leg pain (with woman splaying her fingers apart): Secale
- Back pain but averse to counter-pressure: Nux vomica
- Back pain extends up the back: Gelsemium
- OP baby back pain: Kali carb

- Mother declining direct pressure/heat against her back: Kali carb
- Back pain extends to back and buttocks: Kali carb, Cimic, Pulsatilla, Natrum mur
- All other labour lumbar back pain: Kali carb

Cramps/Spasms

Homeopathic remedies: Rhus tox, Ignatia, Mag phos and Nux vomica

Dehydration

As well as IV fluids:

- Dehydration causing headache: Natrum mur
- Dehydration affecting contractions: Natrum mur/China
- Extreme dehydration: China

Exhaustion (Maternal)

If early in labour, consider an opioid (e.g. pethidine, morphine) to allow the client a break from her contraction pain, to recover her strength.

NATUROPATHY

- Eat food rich in polyphenol micronutrients (instead of sugar), e.g. flaxseed meal, many dried herbs, blackcurrants, capers, plums, olives, many nuts, spinach, red onion, dark chocolate.
- IV fluids and rehydration drinks.

HOMEOPATHY

- Some main remedies: Arsenicum, Carbo veg, Caul and Gelsemium
- General exhaustion with no specific clear symptoms: Kali phos
- From prolonged labour: Arnica/Rescue Remedy
- With aggressive anxiety (and thirst): Arsenicum alb
- With head feeling heavy: Gelsemium
- With being sluggish, difficult and worn out: Sepia
- Physical exhaustion: Fluoric acid
- Mental exhaustion: Phos acid
- Nervous exhaustion: Kali phos
- Dehydration/loss of body fluids exhaustion: China (Cinchona)
- Exhaustion blend of Fluoric acid, Phos acid, Kali phos and China. Can give a sudden extra burst of natural energy to help see the woman through to delivering the placenta. (Aids PPH recovery too for better breastfeeding.) Take 2 drops sublingually during labour-birth when feeling exhausted.

Fear and Shock (Emotional)

NATUROPATHY

- Homeopathy shines brightly as an effective beacon of hope with managing practically all debilitating emotions, however herbalism can also be very useful. Thus, for chronic conditions the woman could benefit from a consultation.
- Essential oils: lavender, ylang ylang, melissa, cedarwood, blue tansy, magnolia, green mandarin, and yarrow,

applied topically (diluted) and diffused.

HOMEOPATHY

- Fear/shock blend for PTSD: Aconite and Opium. Take 2 drops sublingually as required (i.e. when there are extreme surges of intense fear, and as adrenaline support).
- Anxiety remedies: Aconite/Arsenicum alb/Cimic/ Gelsemium/Pulsatilla/Rhus tox
- Fear remedies: Aconite/Cimic/Gelsemium
- Fearful, restless, anxious, labour too quick or fear of death: Aconite
- Anxiety causing restlessness: Rhus tox
- Deep fear stalling labour: Cimic

Nausea and Vomiting

Options instead of, or as well as, anti-emetic drugs.

HOMEOPATHY

- Main nausea and vomiting remedies: Arsenicum alb, Ipecac and Phosphorous
- Fainting (not vomiting): Ferrum phos
- Nausea and vomiting after eating: Nux vomica
- Nausea (unrelieved by vomiting): Ipecac
- Feeling faint especially if cold but needing fanning: Carbo veg
- Nausea and vomiting with faintness, dyspnoea and back pain: Pulsatilla
- Feeling faint with strong ineffectual urge to urinate/pass stools: Nux vomica

Sciatica

Main Homeopathic remedies: Cimic, Coffea, Kali bich, Kali carb and Rhus tox.

Labour-Birth Medical Complexities and Obstetric Complications

Important Note

The following therapies are in addition to the appropriate and timely normal obstetric management of medical emergencies.

Collapse (Maternal)

Post-collapse cold and limp: homeopathic remedy Carbo veg

Author Comment

As a "real-world" pragmatic observation, all post-birth maternal collapses that have occurred within my personal caseload were all some of the rare women who declined a "hot chocolate" beverage drink after their baby was born. For my practice, the hypothesis of hypoglycaemia became such an obvious correlation, I began to *insist* all women have a sugary drink asap after completion of the third stage and control of bleeding – and I've never since had another woman faint.

Convulsions

Obviously an obstetric medical emergency.

Complementary Homeopathic remedies: Apis, Belladonna and Hypericum

Fetal Distress (heartrate concerns)

After maternal position change and emergency delivery considerations.

Homeopathic remedy: Carbo veg and potentially Arnica

Hypersensitivity (Immune system overactivity)

Symptoms such as skin rash, fever and shortness of breath.

Main Homeopathic remedy: Arnica

Hypertension (Maternal)

NATUROPATHY

- If any antenatal history of hypertension, even borderline, consulting with a herbalist/naturopath during the pregnancy can better equip the woman's body for the exertion of childbirth, as can Acupuncture.
- Essential oil: ylang ylang. Dilute and apply to hand palms, feet soles and over the heart, and aromatherapy diffusing into the air. (Woman can also apply the oil to her palms, and inhale from her hands cupped over her nose.)

HOMEOPATHY

- Sudden high BP and acute and flushed face: Belladonna
- High BP and headache and picture of dehydration:

Natrum mur
- High BP with low urine output and proteinuria: Apis

Meconium-stained Liquor

Homeopathic remedy: Carbo veg

Post-birth Urine Retention

Homeopathic remedy for maternal urination delay: Arnica

PPH (Postpartum Haemorrhage/Hypotonic Uterus)

If there is one skill-set a team of midwives/obstetricians can be incredibly proficient in – in fact typically on "auto-pilot" – it is management of a PPH emergency. However, where we collectively remain poorly educated on are prophylactic and cessation options (alongside pharmaceutical oxytocics), and PPH recovery options (alongside blood transfusion).

NATUROPATHY

Herbalism (Western, Indian Ayurvedic and Chinese traditional medicine) all have many treatments to assist PPH recovery.

HOMEOPATHY

Homeopathy especially is useful for post-PPH emotional trauma recovery. But it also has many remedies that can complement obstetric emergency protocols to assist to control bleeding.

Before the PPH:

- Prophylactic for women high-risk for PPH: Arnica

During the PPH:

- Main remedies: Aconitum, Arnica and Caul
- Fear and pounding pulse: Aconite
- Profuse/sudden, hot clots, gushing: Belladonna
- Woman gasping: Carbo veg
- Foul smelling, dark black clots: Carbo veg
- Slowly trickling blood that won't stop: Caul
- Persistent, passive, thin and dark haemorrhage with boggy uterus: China
- Heavy, slow, dark flow with clots: Cimic
- Bright red and not clotting: Ipecac
- Profuse, constant, hot, bright red: Ipecac
- Bleeding worse on moving or lying down: Ipecac
- Bleeding with pain at umbilicus: Ipecac
- With severe back pain: Kali carb
- Dark and oozing/thin blood: Secale
- Fierce contractions then gushing blood: Secale
- Dark blood, no clots, offensive odour, atonic uterus: Secale
- Haemorrhage after RPOC: Pulsatilla

After the PPH:

- Main PPH remedy for Anaemia: China and Ferrum phos
- Main PPH remedy for Laceration: Calendula
- Huge loss of body fluid (especially if collapsed): China
- Exhaustion blend of Fluoric acid, Phos acid, Kali phos and China. Aids PPH recovery for better breastfeeding.

Pre-labour SROM (Spontaneous Rupture of

Membranes) at Term

NATUROPATHY

Obviously consulting with a naturopath at the time of a "term" pre-labour SROM is not always immediately possible. However, a consultation as soon as practical can be beneficial because herbalists do have specific remedies to assist labour contractions to commence.

OTHER REMEDIES UNTIL LABOUR COMMENCES

- Sip homeopathic "birth mix" hourly
- Evening primrose capsules: 4000mg 3 times a day
- Eating spicy food ("activating" the bowels can activate contractions)

PTL (Pre-term Labour)

In general, under 34 weeks everything possible is done by modern obstetric medicine to halt the labour contractions. Whereas at 34–37 weeks the pending arrival of a premature baby is somewhat more accepted. This is where homeopathy in particular may sometimes be the only option to possibly cease the unwanted contractions.

NATUROPATHY

- Obviously consulting with a naturopath at the time of PTL is commonly not logistically possible. However, for a woman who has a history of a premature birth, or a current irritable uterus, she may strongly benefit from a consultation because herbalists do have specific remedies to assist to stop PTL.
- Women who do have a premature newborn can assist

their lactation by taking herbal lactagogues (refer "Breastmilk Under-supply" in Postpartum section).

HOMEOPATHY

- Threatened PTL: Sepia
- Fast PTL: Mag phos
- Sudden and fast PTL: Aconite/Mag phos
- PTL from shock: Aconite
- PTL from trauma: Arnica
- PTL from a twisting fall: Rhus tox
- PTL from fever/infection: Belladonnna
- PTL from pregnancy of multiples: Sepia
- PTL with fast urge to push: Sepia

Pyrexia (Fever)

During labour, in general a temperature over 38°C/100°F *after* administration of NSAID, with or without fetal tachycardia, is cause for an obstetric consultation. Homeopathy with the NSAID may assist the woman's body to return to homeostasis.

HOMEOPATHY

- Main fever remedy: Belladonna
- Woman says she feels hot internally, but is cold to touch: Secale
- Dry heat with glazed expression and flushed face: Belladonna
- With thirst and weakness: Caul
- Sudden high fever: Belladonna

RPOC Retained Products of Conception (Retained Placenta)

If there is an opportunity to consult with a naturopath, herbalism can usually help, and typically something along the lines of slippery elm, or Angelica (Archangelica) tincture is prescribed.

HOMEOPATHY

- RPOC main remedy: Pulsatilla
- With "tearing" lower abdominal pain: Cimic
- With sharp/shooting/cutting pains: Cimic/Sepia/Gelsemium

Shock/Fainting

Main Homeopathic remedies for reanimation: Aconitum, Antimonium tart, Arnica and Carbo veg.

The Postpartum (First Six Weeks Postnatal)

Maternal Wellbeing (Mother)

Recommended Must-haves for All Postpartum Women

- For healthy woman after natural birth: Homeopathic Arnica 4–6 doses a day during the first 48 hours greatly assists internal bruising, inflammation and general recovery. This is especially for long, difficult labours.
- High-quality daily multi-mineral, multi-vitamin supplement
- High-quality omega-3 DHA oil supplement
- HyperCal (hypericum-calendula) cream for all skin healing: sore perineum, C-section/episiotomy incisions, and pending sore nipples
- Consider chewable tablet of vitamin C and zinc (especially if an instrumental/surgical delivery)
- Consider Rosehip Oil for scar healing (especially if C-section or episiotomy)
- Consider a one-month supply of Siberian ginseng to assist in combating the normal sleep-deprivation of the postpartum period (especially if any history of depressive disorders)

After-pains/Postpartum Pains

NATUROPATHY

- Various herbal combinations can be useful – refer to your naturopath/medical herbalist
- Acupuncture, acupressure, warm compresses, massage and pharmaceutical analgesia can also provide relief

- Essential oils: frankincense, geranium and lavender

HOMEOPATHY

- Main routine tincture: Caul
- Severe cramping ("You are cramping my space" emotions): Cuprum
- Unable to tolerate the slightest twinge of discomfort ("Princess" emotions): Platina
- After-pains with severe breaking back-pain ("school teacher timetable" emotions): Kali carb
- Grand multip after-pains: Sabina (or perhaps Sepia or Secale)
- Primarily feeling bruised and sore: Arnica
- Persistent and painful: Secale
- After-pains much worse with breastfeeding: Arnica, Cham and Secale
- After-pains feeling unbearable: Cham and Cimic
- After-pains feeling better with heat/movement (worse with cold): Rhus tox
- Pains with disappointment/resentment: Staphysagria, Sepia and Natrum mur
- After-pains from RPOC: use birth-mix blend, then after MROP (manual removal of placenta) use the uterine cleansing tonics such as Shepherd's Purse (*Thlaspi bursa pastoris)* tincture
- Cramping with blood clots (?RPOC): a blend of Arnica, Hamamelis, Bellis, Hypericum and Staphysagria. Take 2 drops sublingually 3–4 times a day or as required. And/or mix 4–6 drops in cup warm water, shake, and sip throughout the day – especially if recovering from instrumental or surgical delivery.
- Severe after-pains: a blend of Cuprum met, Hepar sulph and Secale. Take 2 drops sublingually 3–4 times a day or

as required. And/or mix 4–6 drops in cup warm water, shake, and sip throughout the day.
- Flushing pains: Belladonna
- Walking/sitting pains: Camphor
- Severe crampy pains: Bellis
- Spasmodic lower abdo pains (esp after long labours): Caul
- Intense groin pains with agitation: Cimic
- Severe pains with irritability: Cham
- Gut (not womb) aches: Cocculus
- Strong pain causing insomnia: Coffea
- Pains causing distress: Cuprum
- Rectum/bladder discomfort (esp right side): Lac caninum
- Pain travelling forward from back to front: Sabina
- Bearing-down pain that radiates upwards: Sepia
- Post C-Section pain: Chamomilla, Arnica, Cuprum and Xanthoxylum

Anaesthesia Recovery

HOMEOPATHY

- Main remedies for anaesthesia unpleasant effects: Opium and Phos
- Post narcotics (pethidine/morphine): Nux vomica, Cham and Rhus tox
- Post epidural: Hypericum, Arnica and Opium
- Post oxytocics: Secale
- Post general anaesthetic: Nux vomica
- Post catheter removal: Staphysagria

Blues and Bonding

(*See also* Depression in this section.)

HOMEOPATHY

- Endless crying: Pulsatilla
- Indifference/poor bonding (suspected PND): Sepia
- General melancholia: Actaea

Breast Engorgement (During First Week)

NATUROPATHY

Essential oils: lavender, geranium and Roman chamomile. Add 3–5 drops to tablespoon fractionated coconut oil and massage onto breasts.

HOMEOPATHY

- Main remedy: Bryonia (and Bellis)
- Slow onset, worse with movement: Bryonia
- Sudden engorgement with breasts throbbing and hot to touch (shower doesn't help): Belladonna
- "Grapevine-looking" red veins and blue lobes: Phytolacca
- Full breasts but milk not flowing: Phytolacca (usually sorted by day 4)
- Shooting pains through the breast: Calc sulph

Breastfeeding – General Wellbeing

NATUROPATHY

Author Comment

I always recommend the woman routinely enjoying a cup of a lactagogue organic nursing tea in the hour before breastfeeding several times a day, to increase hydration and promote a healthy lactation milk flow. The blends typically include herbs such as fennel, fenugreek and anise to help promote lactation, with fragrance such as lavender to ease stress ... and many babies seem to *love* what it does to the flavour of their mother's milk! (I remember feeding my own babies after drinking lactagogue teas and they would look so happy and content, it was as if they would purr if they could while muttering "yum yum yum".)

HOMEOPATHY

- During third trimester for women with history of poor milk supply: Calc phos
- General support: pre-mix such as NaturoPharm's "Milk-Flow" blend of Asafoetida, Bryonia, Calc carb, Phytolacca and Pulsatilla
- Retracted nipples: Sarsaparilla
- "Milk fever" unpleasant mild pyrexia of supply arriving: Arnica
- Fear of painful feeding: Cham, Aconite, Arsenicum alb
- Intolerable painful "empty" feeling when breastfeeding: Borax
- Pain radiating from nipple: Cham, Calendula
- Reducing let-down discomfort: blend mix of Ignatia, Opium and Natrum mur. Take 2 drops sublingually prior to feeding baby, until improvement

Breastmilk Over-supply (at 5–6+ Weeks)

NATUROPATHY

- Teas: sage and jasmine
- Herb: parsley (e.g. tabbouleh)
- Essential oil: apply cold compress of peppermint oil

HOMEOPATHY

To reduce milk-flow: Pulsatilla

Breastmilk Under-supply

(Also refer infant "Failure to Thrive" later in this chapter.)

Note: On most occasions the issue is not low milk production, but actually a poor latch.

NATUROPATHY

- Initially: fennel and blessed thistle capsules (discontinue fennel after 10 days or if it excessively increases urinary output)
- Essential oils: warm compresses of fennel, clary sage and basil

HOMEOPATHY

- Main remedy: Lactuca virosa
- General poor supply: Natrum mur and Aconite
- Increasing supply: Urtica urens and Ricinus communis. Mix 5 drops of both in 50 ml water, then drink 10 ml 3–4 times a day until milk flow established
- Late arrival and diminishing quantity: Asafoetida

24-HOUR MILK SUPPLY BOOST FIX

A great way to rapidly and significantly increase milk supply requires *one* 24-hour commitment:

- *For 24-hours the woman does* nothing *but breastfeed, breast-pump, eat and sleep.*
- *She stimulates her breasts (with breastfeeding or breast-pumping) for a minimum 20–30 minutes every 2-hours during the daytime (and 3-hourly overnight).*
- *She drinks 4 litres of water per 24 hours.*

Typically, this massively and dramatically increases her milk supply.

Caesarean Scar Dehiscence

Additional to normal medical management:

- Increasing magnesium, zinc and protein in diet.
- Properly resting! (Ensuring optimal in-home household helpful support)
- HyperCal lotion several times daily to inhibit infection and stimulate healing.

Catheterization

Main Homeopathic remedies for unpleasant effects from catheterization: Causticum and Staphysagria

Constipation

Refer Antepartum section remedies.

Depression and Anxiety Disorders

Red alert situation — don't dismiss.

NATUROPATHY

- Depression and anxiety disorders can benefit enormously from a private consultation to diagnose cause. Hormone-balancing herbalism remedies, be it Western, Chinese traditional medicine or Indian Ayurvedic treatments – along with dietary advice and time specifically allocated for meditation, yoga or exercise.
- Acupuncture is also very well proven to reduce depression symptoms
- Essential oils: lemon, lavender, frankincense and clary sage

Author Comment

For common new-parenting sleep-deprivation-induced depressive feelings, an over-the-counter central nervous system tonic that naturally boosts serotonin may be all that is necessary to very effectively inhibit the development of full-blown PND. Two personal favorites are:

- *For the mother:* Siberian ginseng. It can also be a highly effective PND prophylactic when taken in the final month of pregnancy for a woman with a history of PND.
- *For the partner:* 5-HTP. Sometimes the partners, also being sleep-deprived, can become even more anxious as a new parent than the woman herself, and this supplement taken at night can effectively ease debilitating over-worrying.

HOMEOPATHY

There are many dozens upon dozens of potential 'best' remedies. Oftentimes, requires consultation with classical homeopath to determine constitutional tincture. Examples:

- Main remedies for depression: Pulsatilla and Sepia
- Main remedy for nervousness and restlessness: Chamomilla
- General melancholia: Actaea
- Severe melancholia: Platina
- With nervousness, drowsiness and constipation: Opium
- With feelings of being abused: Staphysagria
- From birth disappointment of failed high-ideal expectations: Ignatia
- With irritability: Actaea
- With nervousness, restlessness, gloom and sleeplessness: Actaea
- With restless anguish: Arsenicum alb
- With fretful irritability: Merc sol
- With loss of spirits, self-discouragement, self-isolation and hunger: Iodum
- With philosophically worried and aversion to washing/ warmth: Sulphur
- With crossness or fidgetiness: Cham
- With sleeplessness of feeling hot: Aconite
- With anguish, cold skin and/or cold sweats: Verat
- Acute depression and history of large fluid loss: China
- Due to separation from baby: Natrum mur
- Post IUD/stillbirth emotions: Cimic
- PTSD fear/shock blend for traumatic birth/flashbacks: Aconite and Opium. Take 2 drops sublingually as required (i.e. when there are extreme surges of intense fear, and as adrenaline support).

- For chronic PND: consult with classical homeopath for constitutional diagnosis.

Haemorrhage (secondary bleeding)

Medical consultation of course depending on severity.

(Also refer Intrapartum section)

NATUROPATHY

If persists, consult with a herbalist (Western, traditional Chinese medicine or Ayurvedic), who will have many tools that can help.

HOMEOPATHY

- Main secondary PPH remedy: Trillium
- Great loss of body fluids: China
- Emotions increasing bleeding: Thlaspi bursa
- Suspected RPOC: Shepherd's Purse/birth-mix

Haemorrhoids

Refer Antepartum section.

Incontinence

In addition to Kegel pelvic-floor exercises:

HOMEOPATHY

- Incontinence (weak pelvic floor) when coughing/sneezing: Causticum
- Stress incontinence blend: Causticum, Sepia and

Trillium. Take 2 drops sublingually 3–4 times a day. And/ or 4–6 drops in cup of warm water, shake, and sip throughout the day.

- Weak/exhausted pelvic-floor: Gelsemium
- Weak bladder/abdominal muscles: combo of Trillium and Sepia. Take 2 drops sublingually 3–4 times a day. And/or 4–6 drops in cup of warm water, shake, and sip throughout the day.

Insomnia

NATUROPATHY

- 5-HTP (serotonin booster excellent for the *next* night after a previous night of little sleep)
- Melatonin supplements (sometimes treated as a doctor-only hormone prescription)
- Kava supplements
- Magnesium mineral
- Lavender essential oil
- Tea: Valerian root, hops and chamomile
- Passion flower
- Glysine (amino acid)
- California poppy, lemon balm, chaste tree, magnolia bark, jujube
- Tryptophan, ginkgo biloba, L-theanine

HOMEOPATHY

- From anxious apprehension: Gelsemium
- From anxiety: Aconite, Arsenicum alb
- From excitement: Arsenicum alb, Gelsemium
- From pharmaceutical drugs: Cham, Rhus tox, Nux

vomica
- With sleeplessness and restlessness in a nervous person: Actaea
- From busy mind of crowded thoughts and agitation: Coffea
- Drowsy at first then nervous and restless: Opium
- With Neurasthenia (physical and mental exhaustion accompanied by occipital headaches): Xanthoxylum
- With anxious dreams, hot, restless and tossing about: Aconite
- With restless nervousness and twitching: Scutellaria
- With nervous exhaustion and restlessness: Avena sat
- With bounding pulse: Veratrum vir
- Sleeplessness from lack of sleep: Cocculus

Lochia (Unpleasant)

HOMEOPATHY

- Release of clots and flatulence: Nux vomica
- Milky, resembling vaginal discharge: Pulsatilla
- Very dark: Secale
- Thin and foul smelling that lasts too long: Rhus tox
- Foul smelling with bearing-down pains: Sepia, Nux vomica
- Foul smelling with history of traumatic/rapid birth: Aconite
- Offensive, suppressed or insufficient: Sulphur

Mastitis (Breast Infection)

NATUROPATHY (many potential remedies)

- Externally a poultice of grated potato and ginger
- Internally echinacea, zinc and garlic
- With an infection/suspected abscess not settling with antibiotics, also consider dietary advice, boosting immune system, probiotics, and acupuncture
- Essential oils: lavender, patchouli, a citrus blend. Dilute in carrier oil and apply 1–2 drops on breasts.

HOMEOPATHY

- Main remedies: Belladonna, Bryonia and Lac caninum
- Red streaks radiating from the centre: Belladonna
- Engorgement and potential mastitis: Belladonna, Bryonia and Phytolacca blend. Take 2 drops sublingually 3–4 times a day until symptoms reduced. And/or 4–6 drops in cup of warm water, shake, and sip throughout the day.
- Confirmed mastitis: Natrum mur and Calendula
- Threatened abscess: Bryonia (first 48 hours). **If likely abscess forming: Phytolac pyrogen** to draw the pus out; then Hepar sulph to reabsorb it; then Calen to cleanse it
- **Confirmed abscess**: Hepar sulph, Silicea terra and Merc sol
- Topical ointment to abscess incision: HyperCal or Calendula cream

Nipple Trauma (Sore/Cracked)

NATUROPATHY

- Bioptron light therapy
- Nipple shells (not to be confused with nipple shields)

- Hydrogel healing pads
- Essential oils: lavender, geranium and tea tree

HOMEOPATHY

- General routine trauma: HyperCal (or Calendula cream if HyperCal not available) applied topically after every feed (and gently wiped off before feeds – not because it is toxic but simply so baby doesn't find the nipples slippery to latch to)
- Main remedies for fissured nipples and painful breastfeeding: Calendula and Castor equi
- Cracked nipples: Castor equi/Sepia
- Tender and inflamed: Cham
- Too painful to latch: Staphysagria. Sore and cracked: blend of Castor equi and Phytolacca. Take 2 drops sublingually 3–4 times a day to assist with healing, and 4–6 drops in cup of warm water, applied to the nipple after feeding.

Author Comment

My all-time favourite winning combo to effectively treat sore, traumatized nipples is:

- HyperCal cream applied after every feed
- Wearing HydroGel disc-pads between feeds
- Plus, having baby's latch checked by a lactation consultant, or midwife, or friend/family who has successfully breastfed several children.
- After a couple of days, if things are not improving, replace daytime wearing of HydroGel disc pads between feeds with wearing nipple shells (not to be confused

with nipple shields, which generally should only be used by women as temporary assistance with initially flat or inverted nipples).

Perineal/Vulva/Wound Healing

NATUROPATH

- Good diet of micronutrients, especially zinc and garlic, and Echinacea
- Herbalist and acupuncture can be very helpful for speeding healing
- Essential oil: lavender

HOMEOPATHY

- For bruising/trauma/shock: Arnica
- Post instrumental vaginal delivery: Bellis
- Episiotomy healing: Staphysagria and Hypericum
- Post C-section surgery: Bellis (and Arnica, Calendula, Hypericum)
- General trauma/wound mix for perineal discomfort of swelling and bruising. Blend of Arnica, Hamamelis, Bellis, Hypericum and Staphysagria. Take 2 drops on tongue 3–4 times a day as required. And/or add 4–6 drops in cup of warm water, and sip throughout the day.
- Swollen labia: apply diluted Lobelia
- Post C-section stretching/pulling pain discomfort: Staphysagria
- Post C-section keloid scarring: Silica

Author Comment

HyperCal cream is simply amazing for *all* skin healing. The Hypericum relieves nerve pain and the Calendula promotes healing. (Over one eight-year 24/7 caseload of more than 500 women, my clients had *no* postpartum C-section wound or perineal infections, ever, from generous topical use of HyperCal. It is a near-miraculous product. Directions: reapply after each visit to the toilet.)

Phlebitis (vein inflammation)

Red alert for inflamed, swollen, painful veins on arms or legs.

Main complementary Homeopathic remedies: Belladonna and Bryonia

Prolapse

Rectal: Homeopathic Hamamelis, Ruta and Sepia

Uterine: Homeopathic Sepia

Puerperal Sepsis (Uterine Infection)

Pyrexia (fever) of an unknown origin with rigors (shivering/shaking), or known Endometritis *must* always be treated with the utmost seriousness, and receive a specialist obstetric consultation and prompt antibiotics.

NATUROPATHY

- Immune system boost such as Echinacea
- Hot flannels applied to the abdomen can ease symptoms
- Essential oils: clary sage, bergamot, myrrh and Douglas

fir.

HOMEOPATHY

Use in conjunction with medical care-plan management:

- Main sepsis infection remedy: Pyrogenium
- Sudden onset and/or fever: Belladonna
- Slow onset and hot to touch: Bryonia
- Dark, putrid lochia, burning fever and painful after-pains: Secale
- Dry skin, heat, pain, anxiety and restlessness: Aconite
- With an infection diagnosis: Ecchin and Sulphur
- Extreme tenderness, abdominal distension, bloody, slimy discharge: Merc cor
- Sudden stitch and cries of pain (likely nocturnal): Kali carb
- Extreme abdominal tenderness, improved after sleeping: Lachesis
- Pyaemic conditions (eg *Staphylococcus septicaemia*): Pyrogen

Stretch Mark Reabsorption

Main oral Homeopathic remedy: Thiosinaminum

Urinary Retention

Primary Homeopathic Remedies:

- With desire to urinate, and likely distress/anxiety/fear: Aconite
- With urge to urinate, but feeling sore/bruised/injured: Arnica

- Constant dribbling of urine after childbirth: Arnica
- With urgent frequent desire to urinate and occasional small involuntary amounts: Causticum

Uterine Atony (Secondary womb sub-involution)

NATUROPATHY

Prophylactic: after birth continuing to use up whatever supplies of Nature's Sunshine "5-W" are left over from the pregnancy.

HOMEOPATHY

- PPH with Depression (red alert). Main remedies: Ignatia, Kali carb, Kali phos, Natrum mur
- Uterine tonic of and Shepherd's Purse *(Thlaspi bursa)* to assist to cleanse the uterus and relieve after-pains. Mix 5 drops in cup of water. Drink 10 ml 3 times a day until tincture finished.
- Other potentially helpful remedies: Secale, Caul, Cimic, Sepia and Pulsatilla.

When health is absent, wisdom cannot reveal itself, art cannot manifest, strength cannot fight, wealth becomes useless, and intelligence cannot be applied.

Herophilus (335–220 BCE), Greek physician

Neonatal Wellbeing (Newborn)

NOTE. *The use of homeopathic drops officially does not impact the WHO's definition of a baby being "exclusively" breastfed.*

Normal Initial Transition (to Extrauterine Life)

HOMEOPATHY – ROUTINE

To gently assist normal neonatal transition from intrauterine to extrauterine life, the author suggests birth practitioners carry a routine blend tincture with 5 drops each of Aconite, Carbo veg and Opium in teaspoon of cooled boiled water, and administer 2 drops to the newborn as soon as practical, then repeat every 15–20 mins until babe clearly content and blossoming.

ADDITIONAL HOMEOPATHIC BIRTH RECOVERY REMEDIES

Administer to baby as soon as possible after delivery, and for first 4 days:

- Babe appears shocked: Aconite
- Long/traumatic birth: Arnica
- Irritable and shrieking: Cham/Belladonna/Apis/Arnica, and Bach's Rescue Remedy
- Difficult to settle: Arnica/Arsenicum alb/Rhus tox
- Excessive moulding/caput: Arnica
- Bruised head: Arnica
- "Tight shoulders" at birth: Arnica
- Rigorous shoulder dystocia manoeuvres at birth: Arnica and Hypericum alternated

- Quiet and "lifeless": Arnica
- Sticky-eye at birth: Aconite

Cephalohaematoma (Skull Haematoma)

ESSENTIAL OILS

Pure oils helichrysum, geranium and/or fennel. Dilute 1–2 drops in 2 tablespoons fractionated coconut oil and apply sparingly.

HOMEOPATHY

- Initially 'trauma' blend (e.g. Aconite, Arnica and Stramonium)
- If not responding (no reabsorption): Hepar sulph

CMPA (Cow's Milk Protein Allergy)

This is an allergic response (more aptly described as an "oversensitive intolerance") to proteins commonly found in cow's milk. The immune system has an abnormal reaction because it thinks the protein is a threat and goes into attack mode. It is the commonest allergy in young children (roughly about one in 20). Fortunately, most infants outgrow this allergy, usually between three months and three years of age (and almost half in time for ice creams at their first birthday).

Both formula-fed and breastfed babies can be allergic (although chances are significantly lowered in exclusively breastfed babes) – formula-fed babies are allergic to the cow's milk proteins in the formula, and breastfed babies to the dairy products consumed by their mother. Symptoms can show between three-quarters of an hour (rapid onset) to more than 20 hours after ingestion. Although there is no treatment as such, symptoms can be controlled.

Symptoms can appear within the first months of life, or first month of being fed formula. As with all allergies, the body's defence system produces histamines to make the blood vessels dilatate and capillaries secrete, which can cause an itchy, bumpy skin rash (hives), eczema or dermatitis.

SYMPTOMS OF CMPA

- Loose poo (diarrhoea), possibly containing blood
- Mucosa membranes produce extra mucus, which can make baby wheezy and congested with constant sniffles or continual clear runny nose
- Abdominal cramping pains
- Irritable colicky crying
- Vomiting
- Consistent constipation
- Nappy rash
- Nausea or behavioural changes
- Sudden and extremely serious anaphylactic reaction including face, mouth and tongue swelling, making it difficult to breathe. (This is very rare.)

POSSIBLE CMPA REMEDIES

- A classical homeopath identifying the constitutional remedy
- Avoid introducing formula within the first three months, and continue breastfeeding for as long as possible, ideally for at least six months
- If breastfeeding, mother removes all dairy products from her diet, and any other foods that are allergenic

- If formula-feeding, change to a goat's milk formula or hydrolysed hypoallergenic formula, or soy-based formula (however many infants are also allergic to this). It is trial and error.
- Try antihistamine medications (natural or pharmaceutical).
- Make the baby's diet dairy-free once baby is on solids (but a cow's milk protein allergy usually means an infant can still eat beef)
- Put a hot-water bottle or heated wheat bag wrapped in a hand towel or cloth nappy on baby's tummy
- Offer a relaxing pacifier for baby to suckle on to aid digestion
- Consider having baby's constitution analysed by a classical homeopath
- Consider having baby's wellbeing checked by a medical herbalist
- Half or more of CMPA infants go on to develop other hyposensitivity intolerances, such as allergies to soy, eggs, peanuts, citrus fruit and/or inhaled allergens such as pollen.

Colic

Colic is not a disease – it is a temporary physical disorder. Some experts estimate that about 20–25 per cent of babies can suffer a little from colic, but that only about 10 per cent of those (i.e. one in 40–50 babies) are considered severe cases. Other experts estimate that about one in 20 babies suffer from full-blown colic. But either way, it isn't uncommon.

Colic is popularly defined as the 3-3-3 rule: an otherwise healthy infant, crying for more than three hours a day, for more than three days a week, for more than three weeks.

(Colicky babes tend to become particularly inconsolable in the evenings, and typically around the same time every night.)

TRIAL-AND-ERROR REMEDIES FOR COLIC

- If chronically persisting, altering the mother's diet and consulting with a herbalist can potentially provide relief
- Regularly burping baby during feeds
- Removing baby from an overstimulating environment
- Mother checking she isn't "fiddling" with her baby while feeding (e.g. playing with her toes or rubbing her arm). A baby's language is touch, and to her your "fiddling" may be overstimulating, exciting, distracting, and making her tummy uptight.
- A pacifier to suckle may help digestion, as it triggers oxytocin production. The down-side is that the baby could end up swallowing more air.
- Allow the baby to vent some frustration through a little crying, in the hope that it stimulates endorphins
- Feeding baby when the mother's breasts aren't engorged (express a little off if necessary), and feed when the baby is not ravenously hungry
- Feed in a calm, relaxed atmosphere away from loud music and bright lights (though that is good advice for all babies)
- If the baby is formula-fed, swap formula to a brand designed for colicky babies (hypoallergenic). And swap to bottle and teat with special anti-colic valve, such as MAM or Avent.
- Use Dr Harvey Karp's "Five S's": Swaddle, Side, Shush, Swing and Suck
- Warmth can be soothing, so lie baby on a hot-water bottle or heated wheat bag wrapped in a hand-towel or

cloth nappy. Or, fill a little zip-lock plastic bag with warm water and place it on baby's tummy under their nappy. Or, lie baby face down on your lap with a warm hot-water bottle under their belly (not too hot!)

- Massage can be soothing: rub the tummy clockwise, rub the back anti-clockwise (both following the direction of the large intestine's colon); do bicycling motions with baby's legs, give a foot massage
- Try naturopathic and homeopathic remedies, such as Weleda Baby Colic Powder and NaturoPharm Colimed Relief
- Try every brand of infant winding drops
- Try gripe water: typically it contains fennel, and perhaps ginger or dill, and baking soda – but it can also be full of fructose sugar. Variations of gripe waters have been used by mothers for almost 300 years to improve a baby's digestion and relieve colicky crying. (Available in most supermarkets or pharmacies.)
- A little acidophilus and bifidus yoghurt may help baby's digestion – it is also good for the breastfeeding mother to consume
- Antispasmodic prescription-only medicine (e.g. Merbentyl)
- Breastfeeding mother can take essential fatty-acid supplements, or give a formula-fed baby a teaspoon of Efamol daily
- Avoid feeding baby starchy food
- Breastfeeding mothers can try natural teas such as catnip, fennel seed, peppermint, liquorice, chamomile, ginger, or a lactagogue tea-blend such as "Mother's Milk"; and add rosemary to the diet – all can potentially have great tonic effects on a baby
- Consider having baby checked by a neonatal cranial

osteopath
- Consider having baby's constitution analysed by a classical homeopath
- Consider having baby's wellbeing checked by a medical herbalist
- Consider having baby visit an acupuncturist who treats babies
- Avoid repressing crying with over-the-counter sedatives, except occasionally for night-time sleeps (ensuring it doesn't become habitual, otherwise it's like an adult becoming addicted to sleeping tablets)
- Be prepared to try all the crying solutions at the end of my book *Oh Baby*, "Why They Cry" chapter
- In extreme desperation only, take baby for a car ride to help them fall asleep.

HOMEOPATHY

There are hundreds of potential remedies – dependent upon the babe's constitution. If chronically persisting, a strong recommendation for a private consultation with a classical homeopath. A few common examples:

- Main reflux remedies: Nux vomica and Belladonna
- Main colic remedies: Pulsatilla, Sepia, Silica and Cham
- Woken by colic/reflux: Calc sulph
- Due to immature oesophagus (born early/small): Chalcedony
- With distended abdomen and flatulence: Cham/ Pulsatilla/Carbo veg
- Severe colic with flatulence: Trillium
- When baby has extreme irritability and arches their back: Nux vomica
- When baby doubles over, bending forward in pain, and

feels better for passing wind and/or heat on their tummy (e.g. warm hot-water bottle): Mag Phos
- Pain worse with abdominal pressure, and pain comes on gradually and passes gradually: Stannum
- General reflux/colic blend, typically including Nux vomica, Carbo veg, Nat sulph, Calc phos and Dioscorea. Or suggest diluting 5 drops of each in teaspoon pure water, mix well, and administer 2 drops before and after feeds until noticeable improvements.

Conjunctivitis

- 1–2 drops of breastmilk into the eye with each feed
- Blocked Lacrimal Ducts: Massage and Silica
- Main conjunctivitis remedies: Hepar sulph and Pulsatilla (and red flag for Paediatric check)
- Bathing/wiping eye with *very* diluted homeopathic HyperCal tincture, or Chamomile tea (instead of wiping with water)
- Supportive homeopathic oral remedies: Aconite/ Belladonna/Pulsatilla (and red flag for Paediatric check)

Constipation

Diagnosis of neonatal constipation: pebble-like stools that resemble rabbit droppings.

It is completely normal for an exclusively breastfed baby to irregularly produce stools, even up to only once a week – and so long as when it arrives the poo is soft and yellow, then the baby is *not* constipated. (Formula-fed babies should produce stools several times a day.) Constipation is extremely rare in fully breastfeed baby – but more common in a formula-fed baby during summer.

Management: ensure good hydration – check for signs of dehydration

Straining to pass small volumes: homeopathic Nux vomica

Cough

(Also see "Unwell Baby" at the end of this chapter)

Non-pathological short dry cough of newborns: Nux vomica

Cradle Cap

This is the very common seborrhoea (overactive sebaceous glands) condition (also known as *scurfy scalp*). It starts as pink, raised patches of skin on the scalp that become a yellow-brown crust resembling a dry, scaly eczema — not pretty at all.

You can massage the scalp with a vegetable oil or baby moisturizer, leaving it for a few hours until shampooing at bath time and then rubbing it with a soft baby hairbrush — or leave the oil in overnight, then comb or gently pick the dry skin off the next day. Or an old-fashioned remedy is a paste of 2 teaspoons of bicarbonate of soda and 1 teaspoon water rubbed on, left for five minutes and washed off with baby shampoo. (Cradle cap is also common on baby's eyebrows.)

GENERAL REMEDIES

- Essential oil: Geranium
- Mother increasing B-group vitamins in her diet, or

taking a supplement
- Main homeopathic remedy: Graphites

For chronic persistence of cradle cap, it is best to consult with a naturopath, herbalist and/or homeopath who can often produce excellent results.

Failure to Thrive (Low/slow Weight Gain)

This is generally diagnosed as a *term neonate* (i.e. not premature newborn) who has not returned back to their birthweight by day 14 (or by day 21 for a pre-term premature babe). It is important such babies receive a paediatric assessment to rule out anything more sinister than something as simple as a poor latch resulting in low milk transfer.

With *older baby* (more than 6 weeks), FTT (failure to thrive) is generally regarded as consistently gaining less than 100–150g/4–5 oz per week, or 500g per month.

INITIAL CHECKLIST:

- Breastfeeding dyad assessed by a midwife or lactation consultant to confirm effective latch with good milk transfer
- Consider mother's diet may be low in B12
- Assist newborn homeopathically with remedy Calc phos.

Author Comment: MULTI-PRONG "WHOLISTIC" CARE-PLAN FOR FTT

With a good latch and breastfeeding successfully established, then the commonest cause of FTT is poor feeding habits, such as the overstimulated, overtired "snack and snooze" newborn who continually falls asleep on the breast after a short feed of foremilk. (A well-slept baby is hungry and vigorously feeds well.)

Step 1: FIX THE SUPPLY. A newborn with 6–8 urinations per 24 hours can still be struggling to have a generous weight gain. However, consistently 10–12 wet diapers per 24 hours is always a well-fed newborn. The mother may need to: a) slow her daily pace; b) add in a lactagogue tea to her regime; and c) consider the possibility she may have a milk-flow under-supply that needs attention (see earlier in this chapter).

Step 2: FIX THE FEEDS. Mother to do everything she can to maintain her baby's effective latch and productive suckling for as long as possible with every feed, to ensure her baby receives the fat-rich tummy-filling longer-satisfying *hindmilk*. Feeding goal: seeing baby's eyes roll back with the turkey-dinner "I'm so full!" look.

Step 3: FIX THE SLEEP. Parents to self-educate on infant sleep physiology. Strongly recommended to read the "Infant Sleep" chapter of my book *Oh Baby* which details 12 Golden Rules, 12 Magical Secrets and 20 Do's and Don'ts of teaching a baby to become a great sleeper.

Gastro-oesophageal Reflux

Gastro-oesophageal reflux (GOR) is the baby equivalent of heartburn and also goes by the names of Acid Reflux and Acid Indigestion. The immature valve at the top of the infant's stomach, which is supposed to stop contents moving back up the oesophagus from the stomach, is unreliable, then acid-containing milk from the stomach regurgitates back into the oesophagus. GOR often appears at 2–4 weeks of age, and peaks at around 4 months, then typically begins subsiding from around 7 months on, and is usually outgrown by 9–12 months. However, when symptoms are more severe and interfere with the baby's growth, development, respiration and/or cause serious damage such as ulceration (bloody vomits), then the condition is identified as a disease, going from GOR to GORD (gastro-oesophageal reflux disease).

SYMPTOMS OF GOR

- Baby has volcano-like projectile vomits, even out their nostrils. (If there are bloody flecks in the vomit, this should be treated as evidence of GORD)
- Erratic feeding pattern (refusing to feed because of associating feeding with pain, or wanting to constantly feed to neutralize stomach acids with the antacid effects of the milk)
- Latches on to feed, then shortly afterwards turns head away, arching neck or back, even tossing head from side to side
- Fussing or appearing in pain after eating (even up to an hour afterwards)
- Baby is comfortable when upright, but wails when laid down. (This can also be a symptom of colic.)
- Drools excessively
- May be a restless sleeper, being woken by bursts of pain
- Has wet hiccups or wet burps
- Makes choking, gagging, throaty noises; may have sour breath or recurring wheezing or coughing episodes (from the stomach contents entering the back of baby's throat or his lungs)
- Constant swallowing

- Often seems to suffer from respiratory problems (such as colds, chest infections, wheezing and/or sleep apnoea)
- Poor weight gain.

Note: *An overfed baby can commonly be misinterpreted as a baby with reflux. (There is also a condition called "silent reflux" when there is no vomiting.)*

TRIAL-AND-ERROR REMEDIES FOR REFLUX

- Osteopathy (especially cranial) can produce miraculous results.
- Infant massage techniques can also be beneficial
- Essential oils: lemon, fennel, star anise, marjoram, bergamot, ylang ylang. Dilute 1–2 drops of essential oil in 2 tablespoons fractionated coconut oil and massage a small amount gently on stomach and back.
- Herbalist's special mix of fennel and catnip
- Breastfeeding is strongly preferred over formula, because breastmilk is a natural antacid, is more rapidly digested, and is more intestine-friendly and produces softer poos
- If breastfeeding, take lactation herbs to "thicken" your breastmilk; if formula-feeding, swap to a thickened formula.
- If formula-feeding, the teat hole should permit milk droplets to flow at a too-fast-to-count-the-drips rate, but not "pour" out
- Because swallowing air aggravates reflux, burping during and after feeds can make good sense – infant winding drops may also help
- Giving more frequent feeds of say half as much, twice as often – but, to avoid instilling negative snack-and-

snooze habits, not routinely encouraging feeds less than two-hourly

- Allow half an hour of quiet time after feeds
- Use infant antacid barrier drops such as Gaviscon or Mylanta
- Position baby semi-upright during the day, including during feeds, so that gravity can assist to keep the food down — especially after feeding. (Lying flat on the back can be very aggravating to reflux.)
- Elevate the head-end of baby's bed on an angle (about 30 degrees) and sleep baby on his *left side* enabling the gastric inlet to be higher than the outlet. (Using an abdominal sleep-wrap or baby back-support pillow to stop the baby sliding down, or rolling onto their stomach.)
- Avoid leaving baby sitting in forward positions with a curved spine for long periods (such as hunched in a car-seat or in a pushchair)
- Avoid treating baby with decongestants (which dry their mucus production)
- Warmth on baby's tummy can assist, e.g. a hot-water bottle or heat-pack wrapped in a cloth nappy
- Gentle tummy massage may help
- A pacifier to suckle on may help digestion, as it triggers oxytocin production and stimulates saliva production which can ease reflux irritation. (The down-side is that the baby could end up swallowing more air.)
- Consider having baby checked by a neonatal cranial osteopath
- Consider having baby's constitution analysed by a classical homeopath
- Consider having baby's wellbeing checked by a medical herbalist

- Not encouraging a formula-fed baby to become too "bonny" – obesity can aggravate reflux
- In severe cases, try a prescription-only infant acid-blocker (e.g. Losec or Zantac) at night-time (to reduce stomach-acid production)
- In severe cases, request a prescription-only, prokinetic motility medicine to increase the muscle tone of the lower oesophageal sphincter muscle
- Because crying increases intra-abdominal pressure, it is not possible for a reflux baby to "cry out" an attack of GOR
- Babies with GORD are high-needs babies requiring intensive parental care. Attachment parenting (such as the mother wearing a baby sling) may be beneficial.
- Severe reflux at four months old with suboptimal weight gain is a valid excuse to get on with introducing rapidly digestible solid foods (which may stay down more easily than liquid)
- Most babies show significant improvements once they can maintain an upright posture (e.g. sitting and standing).

HOMEOPATHY

There are hundreds of potential remedies – dependent upon the baby's constitution. If chronically persisting, the strong recommendation is for a private consultation with a classical homeopath. A few common examples of remedies:

- Main reflux remedies: Nux vomica and Belladonna
- Main colic remedy: Cham
- Woken by colic/reflux: Calc sulph
- Due to immature oesophagus (born early/small): Chalcedon

- With distended abdomen and flatulence: Cham/Pulsatilla/Carbo veg
- Severe colic with flatulence: Trillium
- When baby has extreme irritability and arches their back: Nux vomica
- When baby doubles over, bending forward in pain, and feels better for passing wind and/or heat on their tummy (e.g. warm hot-water bottle): Mag Phos
- Pain worse with abdominal pressure, and pain comes on gradually and passes gradually: Stannum
- General reflux/colic blend, typically including Nux vomica, Carbo veg, Nat sulph, Calc phos and Dioscorea. Or suggest diluting 5 drops of each in teaspoon pure water, mix well, and administer 2 drops before and after feeds until noticeable improvements.

Group-B-Strep Exposure

For neonates of a Group B Strep-positive mother, the tincture Antimonium tart is the number one remedy strongly recommended by homeopaths to be given prophylactically to the newborn immediately at birth to prevent RDS (respiratory distress syndrome). Then given 3–4 times a day for the next three days (depending upon the birth scenario, perhaps slightly longer).

Heat Rash

- Rash feels hot to touch (not the entire baby): homeopathic tincture Belladonna
- Heat spots: homeopathic tincture Apis
- Caused from indirect sunlight warmth: homeopathic tincture Natrum mur

Jaundice

Jaundice is common and usually only physiological. Dependent on local protocol, in general any of the following instances confirm pathological jaundice and require paediatric consultation:

- Any jaundice within first 24 hours (this is potentially very serious)
- SBR (bilirubin blood test) >250µmol/L in second 24 hours
- SBR >300µmol/L on days 3–14
- Jaundice visible or SBR >150µmol/L beyond 2 weeks old in a term neonate (or 3 weeks old in a pre-term neonate).

FOR PHYSIOLOGICAL JAUNDICE (and to support medical care-plan of pathological jaundice)

- Constitution consultation with classical homeopath
- Consultation with herbalist (Western, Ayurvedic or Chinese)
- Vitamin E prescription from naturopath
- Jaundice from traumatic birth: Aconite
- If prolonged labour and/or excessive bruising: Arnica
- If mother had pharmaceutical drugs during the pregnancy/birth: Nux vomica
- If baby excessively fussy: Cham
- Jaundice appears acutely/suddenly: Aconite
- If baby lethargic with sluggish bowels: Chelidonium
- If baby irritable and constipated: Lycopodium

Lactose Intolerance (Lactase Deficiency)

Lactose intolerance (also known as lactase deficiency) is a sensitivity to the carbohydrate content in milk from mammals – in other words, an intolerance (inability) for the baby to efficiently break down the lactose sugar within milk, due to their low levels of lactase enzyme production.

It is rare for children to be completely lactose intolerant (i.e. rare to produce extremely low levels of lactase enzymes), so this has tended to be an over-diagnosed condition. However, it is estimated that over half of all babies experience some small degree (for say 1–2 weeks) of lactase deficiency at some stage within their first five months.

To break down lactose, the baby's digestive system provides the enzyme lactase, but if it doesn't, or if there is not enough lactase, fermentation in the large bowel (colon) eventually breaks down the lactose. However, that bacterial fermentation causes side effects.

SYMPTOMS OF LACTOSE INTOLERANCE

- Watery acidic diarrhoea (poo can even be frothy)
- Swollen, bloated abdomen
- Excessive farting
- Stomach cramping, pain that causes crying
- General irritability
- A rumbling stomach.

Note: *Lactose intolerance does not cause vomiting.*

CAUSES OF LACTOSE INTOLERANCE

- A baby does not produce lactase – extremely rare except

in Scandinavia. This is a low-weight, dehydrated and very unwell baby.

- A baby produces levels of lactase that are lower than normal – this is rare in Caucasians/Europeans, but more common in darker-skinned races around the world. It commonly occurs after weaning, and before the age of six.
- A baby who is low in iron can have difficulty with lactose digestion.
- Antibiotics or a parasitic infection (e.g. giardia) can temporarily reduce the baby's lactase levels.
- An episode of gastroenteritis (serious vomiting or diarrhoea) can cause an infant's lactase levels to drop for 1–8 weeks.

POSSIBLE REMEDIES FOR LACTOSE INTOLERANCE

A mother's diet will not affect her breastmilk's consistent levels of lactose. But, it is important to ensure the baby gets all the hindmilk because the fat content aids with the digestion (in other words, make sure the first breast is empty before offering the other breast).

- Delay weaning: breastmilk contains lactase enzymes that help the infant's digestion.
- Space breastfeeds out to at least three-hourly, to avoid the baby snack-feeding on foremilk.
- With formula-fed babies, swap to a lactose-free formula.
- Try lactase drops.
- Once infant is off breast or formula, full-fat milk is better than low-fat varieties. Avoid food containing skim-milk powders.
- Heated milk foods such as custard, milk puddings and warm milk tend to be more tolerable than cold or non-

cooked dairy products.

- Fermented dairy products such as cheeses, butter and yoghurt are usually reasonably well tolerated; and the Swiss cheeses Gruyère and Emmental are practically lactose-free.

Meconium Exposure/Aspiration

For meconium-exposed neonates: the homeopathic tincture Antimonium tart is the number one remedy given prophylactically to the newborn immediately at birth to support to prevent RDS (respiratory distress syndrome). Then given 3–4 times a day for the next three days (depending upon the birth scenario, perhaps slightly longer for thick meconium). For active MAC (meconium aspiration syndrome) RDS, also use Antimonium tart as above.

Nappy Rash

The topic of nappy rash can be a bit of a hornet's nest due to the vast array of remedies available. But normally, if the rash is shiny, red and flat, it is probably a case of ammonia dermatitis burns. As a personal recommendation, Curash™ baby talc powder or a dust of cornflour is great to sprinkle on where a bit of redness has appeared. And an ointment blend of zinc oxide and castor oil can be a good protective barrier cream – but don't use it all the time, just overnight, as necessary.

If the nappy rash has turned into red bumpy pimples (or perhaps even with water-blister pustules), it is probably the fungal infection *Candida albicans* (thrush), which initially thrives in the warm, moist skin creases then spreads outwards, creating a red, raw rash. [My absolute favourite remedy for angry nappy rash is a layer of HyperCal (hypericum-calendula) cream on the skin, then a layer of Mustela® barrier cream (applied so thickly you cannot see the skin).]

If using cloth nappies, avoid using harsh detergents or ammonias by washing in a mild soap. And avoid using plastic-lined disposable nappies or plastic over-pants, as these make for a rather sweaty environment.

Weleda nappy rash cream and NaturoPharm nappymed ointment are also useful in both situations, as can be aloe vera gel, especially as preventatives.

My personal plea to all mothers is to try natural treatments, including homeopathy, before getting into the prescription-only steroid-type medications. But one of the very best and cheapest cures for nappy rash is at least half an hour a day of naked time.

ESSENTIAL OIL

- Lavender: dilute 1–2 drops in 2 tablespoons fractionated coconut oil and apply a small amount topically
- For chronic, stubborn nappy rash, a naturopathic consultation can assist to determine if the maternal diet or poor infant digestion is contributory.

HOMEOPATHY

- Main remedies: Calb carb, Calendula and Medorrhinum
- For raw, red, sore nappy rash: Staphysagria
- For raised, red and moist nappy rash: Rhus tox
- For "tight", swollen nappy rash: Apis

- For chronic, stubborn nappy rash, a homeopathic consultation can assist to determine if it is constitution related
- For severe nappy rash, it is said bathing the baby in their own urine can assist (urine is sterile – and it is the non-sterile *stools* that tend to manifest nappy rash).

Nasal Congestion

- Saline nasal spray drops
- Mist humidifier or steamy bathroom air
- Nasal aspirator
- Main Homeopathic remedies: Calc carb, Kali bich and Lycopodium

Over-tired Newborn (Over-stimulation)

The commonest reasons a term healthy neonate is not feeding well or not sleeping well is because they are *over-tired* (from being *over-stimulated*). The easiest ways to prevent this are:

- Parents being *extremely vigilant* to monitor for the universal infant Tired Signs (because newborns can go from tired to over-tired in 10 minutes).
- Parents intentionally keeping the newborn at home until they are over 5 weeks *and* over 5 kg (or longer), where their air temperature is consistently a thermally-neutral environment; and where their baby is receiving through breastmilk the antibodies for their environment's antigens (germs).
- Bearing in mind the neonate has been in a gentle low-stimulation environment for 9 months prior to birth, the

parents intentionally create a low-stimulation environment for the first 6+ weeks after birth (based on their baby's estimated due date, not birth date), where the visual stimulation is limited to subtle palettes (i.e. TV not on all day); and where the auditory stimulation is limited to gentle talking and easy-listening music (a newborn does not need complete silence to sleep well).
- Diffusing the essential oils of lavender, ylang ylang, lemon, sandalwood and/or the diluted oil massaged into the newborn's feet.
- Diluted drops of the homeopathic remedy Coffea.

Posseting ("Spilly Baby")

Routinely misinterpreted as vomit, this is a baby spilling milk with wind at the end of a feed, as a sort of drool. It is nothing to worry about – it's the baby version of a barfy burp. Posseting usually starts to sort itself out by six months of age, and is usually gone before their first birthday. Main homeopathic remedy: Carbo veg

PPROM (Pre-term Pre-labour Rupture of Membranes)

For newborns with a history of PPROM, administer homeopathic Antimonium tart to baby as soon as practical after delivery, and for first 4 days.

Pyrexia (and Temperature Instability)

Main homeopathic remedies for fever:

- From fever: Belladonna, Bryonia and Gelsemium

- From climate temperature: Calc fluor

(Also see "Unwell Baby" further below.)

Respiratory Distress Syndrome

Refer Meconium Exposure/Aspiration remedies.

Resuscitation Recovery

With baby having a history of low APGAR scores requiring emergency intervention, the following homeopathic tinctures can assist recovery dependent on the baby's *appearance at the time* of resuscitation management. (Administer as soon as practical after delivery and for first four days.)

- Hot, purple, weak heartbeat: Aconite
- Hot red face and staring motionless, rest of body cold: Belladonna
- Pale and feeble responses: Arsenicum alb
- Breath struggling after difficult birth: Arnica
- Low responsivity (and mother large PPH): China
- Low responsivity (and heavy meconium): Carbo veg
- ?Neurological trauma: alternate Arnica and Belladonna

Thrush (Oral)

Instead of, or as well as, medical antifungal drops, the primary homeopathic remedy is Borax – a few drops diluted in boiled cooled water and "swished" around baby's mouth 2–3-hourly.

Traumatic Delivery (e.g. Instrumental)

After birth, use homeopathic fear/shock remedies: e.g. Aconite and Opium

TTN (Transient Tachypnoea of the Newborn)

Abnormally rapid breathing in a very new baby requires a *prompt* paediatric consultation for medical management. Plus supportive homeopathic remedy: Antimonium tart.

Umbilicus (Bellybutton)

Cord flare: umbilical stump red, inflamed, or smelly, or slow to heal: homeopathic oral Calendula and topical HyperCal cream.

Umbilical Hernia: neonate needs paediatric referral. In the meantime, homeopathic remedies Nux vomica or Natrum mur can assist to reduce any newborn discomfort; Calc fluor to assist healing; Trillium pend if abdominal muscles separated.

Unhappy Disposition (consistently crying)

The commonest reason a *brand-new baby* is being incredibly irritable and latching poorly (as if they keep losing their focus), many of us believe, is likely simply a *bad headache*. I have witnessed this as being especially common in babies who received an instrumental delivery by forceps or ventouse.

And the other commonest cause an infant of any age is not feeding well or not sleeping well is because they're *overtired* from being *over-stimulated*. It can be hugely helpful to new mothers to know newborn Tired Signs and have information on the *physiology* of infant sleep (such as accessing the free Infant Sleep articles on the www.motherswise.com website).

As author I also strongly recommend encouraging all "term" newborns don't routinely leave their home environment until they are *over 5 weeks old* (based on due date or birth date, whichever is the later) *and over 5 kg weight* (11 lb). New parents unskilled in neonatal body/sign language tend to use the "winging it" strategy of offering breastfeeding as their go-to first solution to all their newborn's cries. This author suggests new mothers also request their own copy of the *Why They Cry* guide available from www.motherswise.com.

Special Note. Women with postpartum anxiety/depression are well understood to potentially perceive their infant crying as being of significantly greater concern than a mother without PND. So, it is important all mothers know it is completely normal for newborns to communicate through crying for 1–2 hours per 24 hours. Additionally, around 40 per cent of babies naturally have an "angel baby" or "good as gold" nature; and around 40 per cent naturally have a "grumpy" or "difficult to please" personality (and this does not mean the baby is not content or not thriving). The other 20 per cent have personalities that lie somewhere in-between.

ESSENTIAL OILS

To calm: an essential oil "grounding" or "serenity" type blend of frankincense and/or vetiver massaged on the back of the neck, shoulders and bottom of the feet.

Before sleep: essential oil "protective" type blend on the bottom of baby's feet.

HOMEOPATHY

For intense irritability: Apis

For incessant pained crying (headache?): depending on likely root cause, use fear/shock blend (e.g. Aconite and Opium) and/or trauma mix (e.g. Aconite, Arnica and Stramonium).

Unwell Baby (Reasons to Visit a MD)

- A 0–6-week-old with a temperature of 38°C (100°F) or over (a fever). Undress a layer of clothing, and seek urgent medical advice
- A 6-weeks to 3-month-old with a temperature of 38°C (100°F) or over (a fever). Give infant paracetamol (acetaminophen), undress a layer of clothing, and seek prompt medical advice, especially if infant *looks* unwell.
- An over-3-month-old with a temperature of more than 38.5°C half an hour after having paracetamol (acetaminophen), or with continually high temperatures for more than a day. NB: Mild fevers are generally viral, however temperatures higher than 38.9°C can potentially be a serious bacterial infection.
- Troubled, difficult breathing: call an ambulance – *perform CPR if breathing stops*
- Convulsions, seizure fits: call an ambulance (simple fever convulsions are generally not associated with an increased risk of serious infection but still best to get a prompt medical assessment)
- Hard to arouse, unresponsive, lethargic, droopy, floppy, or apathetic – seek urgent medical advice
- Meningism (meningitis-like symptoms such as an unusually high-pitched cry, fever, or possible bulging fontanelle) – seek urgent medical assessment
- Petechial rash (tiny, round, red-brown-purple spots that are flat to touch and may appear in clusters and *don't* lose their colour when you press on them) – seek ***urgent*** hospital consultation
- Crying and listless for no apparent reason
- Breathing with grunting or wheeziness (possible asthma)

- Loud, dry or wheezy cough
- Unusually pale, ashen complexion
- Irritable with swollen abdomen or severe abdominal tummy pain
- Dehydration (e.g. dry lips, dry tongue, sunken fontanelle, lack of tears, reduced wet nappies, e.g. no urine output in 8 hours)
- Poos that are consistently green (may be gastroenteritis) – the occasional guacamole-coloured stool is no concern
- Poos with blood or pus-like mucus in them
- Bad-smelling poo from a breastfed baby (it should smell sweet)
- Diarrhoea lasting longer than 8 hours
- Diarrhoea with vomiting
- Refusing several feeds in a row
- Is upset by his head, neck or ears
- Abnormally low temperature (e.g. 34–36°C, 93–97°F)
- Runny nose with a fever or persistent cough, or looking lethargically sick, or sleeping a lot more than usual. Runny noses are typically very common for older babies because experiencing little colds can frequently occur. However, with small babies having a blocked nose can impact their breathing and feeding (saline nasal drops can give relief) – and seek a medical opinion in timely manner.
- Unusual rash, or strange lump
- Cradle cap that spreads or gets infected
- Yellow or green vomit (containing bile) or blood-stained vomit
- Vomiting for several hours (i.e. more coming out than going in) with a lower threshold tolerance the younger the baby is
- One eye pupil that doesn't change position

- Or anything else the parents are feeling concerned about – it's natural and normal for first-time mothers especially to feel anxious – they are not being neurotic, and they should never be made to feel they should apologize to medical staff for "wasting their time".

Note: If a baby's behaviour demonstrates wellness then this can generally be regarded as a health indicator. For example, if they are vigorous, alert, responsive, not distressed, and feeding satisfactorily, then that is a good sign that any medical assessment is not quite so urgent. However, if a baby is unusually lethargic, has changed to a consistently weak-sounding cry, or just appears sick or unwell, then always treat that more seriously by seeking prompt medical assessment.

Afterword

Surely, it is truly time overdue, that the allopathic automatic-kneejerk lecturing on the potentially 'toxic harmful risks' to pregnant women of self-medicating herbalism, needs to finally realise that the vast majority are actually seeking professional advice from qualified naturopathic practitioners.

Message from the Editor, Kathy Fray
IMHC Research e-Journal, 22 September 2019

Where We've Been

Unless your head is buried in sand, we can all agree that globally our obstetric delivery (versus natural birth) rates in the developed world are way too high – and for many years the increased "emergency deliveries" have stopped corresponding with improving outcomes statistically. Quite the opposite in fact.

At the same time, in universities around the world, our midwives are being formally trained on qualifications being based almost solely on the *science* of midwifery, and in this author's opinion we have lost confidence with some of our competence in the *art* of midwifery, such as being routinely skilled in holistic third-trimester traditional remedies (which midwifery has used since time immemorial) to tone the womb, soften the cervix, naturally induce term labour, and gently augment unproductive contractions.

However, when we ask any self-employed case-loading midwife in the West who has a C-section rate that is consistently low, *how* her women have such high chances of experiencing a beautiful, natural, non-traumatic birth, you nearly always find her birth-kit laden with holistic, naturopathic tools and homeopathic resources. Yet these midwives are rarely honoured, even amongst their own collegial peers. Instead they typically experience ostracism, being shunned as radical fringe extremists (particularly by senior obstetric colleagues). Yet they are just doing their traditional job – typically with excellent statistical outcomes to prove it.

A rare few, like Ina May Gaskin, have managed to be celebrated while straddling the divide between 20th-century alternative hippiedom and 21st-century mainstream medicine (even though we still see obstetricians rarely going for the Gaskin Maneuver first with shoulder dystocias). The culture of ingrained habits can be hard to enlighten, on many levels.

Continually these days still, many midwives who publicly extol the virtues of herbal remedies and vibrational tinctures can still find themselves cold-shouldered and blacklisted, sadly oftentimes by their own kind. This is *not* okay, people. This carnivorous devouring-our-own needs to stop!

Another sad fact contributing to the rampant hospitalization, over-medicalization of childbirth is the reality that most birthing suite doctors today (both obstetricians and paediatricians) often never see all those many, *many* babies that are beautifully, stunningly birthed in homes and primary-care locations.

Yet every day these same doctors do routinely see the traumatized babies who have been yanked out, sucked out, or cut out, and the consequential sequelae of neonatal (and maternal) morbidity complications. But somehow everyone accepts seeing so many neonates with low APGAR scores due to their prolonged augmented labours and dramatic obstetric deliveries – it is as if health professionals rarely question how those abnormal outcomes came to be so prolific.

At the same time, I don't really begrudge obstetricians losing touch with natural labour and normal birth, because for most of these highly trained doctors, "physiologically normal" hasn't been "their normal" for a long, long time. They have become the experts of oxytocin-induced labours and complicated "save the day" deliveries. Consequently, of course their faith in normality has become skewed – how can it not?

However, I do so dream that every 2–3 years, as part of obstetricians' ongoing education, they would be required to include a month with rural midwives in primary-care – away from their secondary/tertiary care hospital facilities – upskill/re-skill their ability to hands-off oversee the care of "natural labour", to remind themselves how most women's bodies are beautifully capable to powerfully give birth normally and safely – in fact most times far more safely than employing their plethora of unnecessary interventions. (When there are no obstetricians left on a birthing suite who feel confident with their competence to handle a multip breech vaginal birth, well, that is just a sad day – and a very real reflection of the culture of many of today's modern hospitals.)

Although the need for obstetric intervention on occasion can of course be black and white, we also all know that both midwives and obstetricians spend *much* of their time operating in "various shades of grey".

We all know ... with midwifery care we must not normalize

what is abnormal. And with obstetric care we must not abnormalize what is normal.

However, a tide is turning. The groundswell has started.

Midwives and doulas have had enough!

Women have had enough!

And refreshingly, holistically-minded obstetricians have had enough, too.

Where We Are Now

Right now in the world there are increasingly generous amounts of authors writing on general Integrative Medicine, and that is a very good thing, driven by the public's demand for holistic health wellness.

However, there remains a dearth of authors writing on the holistic integrative medicine specialty area of *perinatal health* (i.e. naturopathic wellbeing of pregnancy-birth-postpartum-newborn). And although most expectant women during pregnancy are healthy, the fact remains *they are never of their normal health.*

Subsequently, as founding director of IIMHCO (International Integrative Maternity HealthCare Organization), right from its inception I realized, in fact, that *so few* modern books have been written on the topic of integrative medicine for maternal/fetal/neonatal health and wellness, that the specialty didn't even have its own "name" (!) – even though it has existed as a specialty for *thousands of years*. So, one of the first things we did was coin a term to give it a title:

However, today lots of exciting groundbreaking cutting-edge work is being done within this area of medicine. For example, preconception epigenetics and pregnancy nutrition metagenetics are topics currently right at the forefront of scientific research.

At the same time, there are also many ancient traditional texts on herbalistic health during the maternity journey, which modern therapists continue to refer to, especially within traditional Chinese medicine, Indian Ayurveda medicine, and Western herbalism. But despite the *enormous* amounts of anecdotal evidence, often over hundreds and thousands of years, modern allopathic medicine continues to demand their empirical double-blind randomized controlled trials on herbalism and homeopathy.

However, there is more than a slight problem with such a demand:

Who the heck is going to fund all these RCTs?

Certainly not naturopathic medicine – it survives on tiny margins. And certainly not Big Pharma – because they can't earn royalty income from any molecule found naturally in nature. Plus, as we are vibrational beings using vibrational therapies, how does empirical science even begin to efficiently quantify such individualized constitution-based body-mind-spirit healing? They are speaking two different languages ... it is as non-sensical as demanding a Chinese dictionary be written using only English words.

So, then we turn to our naturopathic pharmacological experts who study natural medicine pharmacodynamics (how medicine affects the body) and pharmacokinetics (how the body affects the medicine). But this research is still only scratching the surface to creating an evidence-based approach that Western medicine would pay any credence to as confirming efficacy of natural medicine during the maternity journey because herbs have multiple constituents. (Big Pharma will generally only be motivated to investigate herbal remedies when they believe there is potential to synthesize a royalty-earning equivalent molecule to those found in nature.)

And at the same time, as midwives and obstetricians, we are completely burying our head in the sand too if we believe holistic integrative medicine is not being sought by women worldwide, mainly surreptitiously. Massive evidence continues to pile up of how pregnant women trust their traditional herbalist and question their modern doctor ... it is like we are collectively, as mothers, part of some modern underground resistance, who are insisting on taking charge of their own pregnancy and labour wellbeing, naturopathically.

For example, IIMHCO's Integrative Maternity HealthCare research e-Journal is aware of more than twenty significant research studies focusing on the prevalence of maternal use of prenatal herbs, with the average clandestine usage being around two-thirds of all women globally.

Where We Need to Be

Dear people, it is an absolute *total joke* that some within obstetric medicine (not all) continue believing women believe obstetric medicine to be their "be all and end all" as the best maternity healthcare management available. Some still do. But increasingly, many women do not – not any more. The reputation of obstetric medicine is justifiably under serious question in many Western countries, especially its deeply entrenched one-shoe-fits-all mentality to "throw in the epidural, strap on the CTG, and crank-up the oxytocin" … and if things fail to progress acceptably along Friedman's Curve, then save the day with a heroic emergency obstetric delivery with commentary that ensures the woman feels like you just "saved her baby's life". Thankfully, unlike the compliant mothers in the 1950s and 1960s, our millennials are questioning such medical mentalities – and so they must!

And as front-liners at the coalface, we too as Birth Practitioners, *have* to *stop* respecting *only* empirical scientific evidence and its infamous double-blind trials as being the "be all and end all" to our own "best practice". Of course they *are* of relevance, but they are not the only evidence of relevance.

Science is now admitting its defective capacities to quantify a human's triadic strength of body-mind-spirit, especially with childbirth, which is such a primally raw interconnectedness of the physiological body, the intellectual mind and the soulful spirit.

Many of us (most of us?) are wanting to swing the medical model's pendulum back to a middle path, of formally, officially, and intentionally evolving global maternity healthcare systems into the art of the holistic integrative paradigm openly embracing *perinatal integrative medicine* within the science of gynaecological, midwifery and obstetric healthcare wellness, instead of relying solely on allopathic modern medicine as being the "God" of all perinatal wisdom.

Surely, for all students being formally taught midwifery and obstetrics, basic IMHC skills need to fundamentally become as natural and normal as the natural and normal births we all strive for our clients to experience. Midwives, worldwide, need to reclaim our roles, not just as guardians protecting the *science* of normal birth, but also as custodians defending the *art* of natural labour. And obstetricians, worldwide, need to reclaim their Hippocratic Oath to *first do no harm*.

At IIMHCO, we believe as birth practitioners we all need to proactively expand our circle of those from whom we wish to seek knowledge, to break down the blockades that divide us, and to defeat the tribalism barriers of collegial academia ideology. It's all doable!

Our society with its free speech, open enquiry, and rational debate, does tend to push us in a *moral* direction, in particular, the whole undercurrent that we call humanism, which almost sounds banal and dreary and treacly-sweet nowadays, simply because it has become second nature to us. But over the entire course of human history, our current societal freedoms would have been a radical idea.

Today's enabling of autonomous self-determination and independent liberty, and our clientele's online access to Dr Google and Dr YouTube, expands all our capacities for broad-spectrum thinking. And this, together with our more rational tolerant ethos, is, I believe, making us more holistically minded than ever before. We *are* heading in the right direction. The progress is just slower than a lot of us desire (and faster than a lot of others would prefer).

Should obstetricians share teachings with midwifery students? Of course! Do they? Not a lot. Habitually, it's left to midwives to teach midwifery students.

Should midwives share teachings with obstetric students? Of course! Do they? All the time. Usually because we're so acutely aware the doctor's first-hand obstetric experiences of "normal" will be so limited during their training.

Should our maternity-specializing medical herbalists and homeopaths share teachings with midwifery and obstetric students? Of course!

Do they? Not often. Typically, obstetric junior doctors would never ever attend a lecture on perinatal integrative medicine, and midwifery students may attend the occasional talk by a visiting naturopathic practitioner.

If we are to build a functionally robust integrative maternity healthcare system, we must also all strenuously avoid demonizing another modality of practice therapy such as verbosely regarding them as some ostracized lower-caste pseudo-medical unequal.

Instead, we need to start intentionally and righteously – because it *is* our *right* – aspiring to an insightful merging of ancient remedies with synthetic Big Pharmaceutical; holistic midwifery with medical obstetrics; with us all willing to open our minds – including fully respecting the centuries of accumulated naturopathic anecdotal evidence.

It's about us as maternity healthcare practitioners actively encouraging our women to focus *physically* and *mentally* on pregnancy wellness naturopathically; and to focus *emotionally* and *spiritually* on spontaneous childbirth normalcy.

If our women want *normal health* – then we need to centre them on *natural wellness*.

And if our women want *normal birth* – then we need to centre them on *natural labour*.

But if you are reading this book, then likely we are already on the same page. And right now, at this very moment, you and I are creating history – we are changing the paradigm.

So be proud!

Namaskar,

Kathy Fray

Midwife | Author | MothersWise MD | IIMHCO Founder

Author Postscript

And what of me? Do I walk the walk, or just talk the talk? I felt it was only reasonable I provide you with the stats of my own personal caseload as a self-employed midwife:

Demographics:

- 50% immigrants (English second language)
- 45% primips (first birth)
- 40% advanced maternal age (35–45 years)
- 40% pre-existing medical conditions

Outcomes:

- Average primip active labour: 3–4 hours
- Average multip active labour: 1–2 hours
- Less than 20% epidurals (primarily for C-sections and occasional inductions)
- 40% primary-care birth centre or home birth (only available for healthy, non-complex pregnancies)
- 60% secondary-care hospital labour and birth
- 85% of labours resulting in vaginal births
- 90% fully exclusive breastfeeding at one-month discharge
- Virtually *no* postnatal depression

But why such good statistics for frankly less than an optimal caseload of demographics? The answer, I believe, is really simple:

Advance childbirth education antenatally
& *Partus preparatus* naturopathy

A Reflection on Epidurals

NOTE: As author, I am not anti-epidurals. They absolutely have their place within obstetric medicine. However, I am fervently anti women being unaware of the consequences of their decision to opt for an epidural purely for the purpose of pain management.

The WHO (World Health Organization) advocates around 10–15 per cent of women's babies should be delivered by C-section, which predominantly should be the women with significant obstetric complexities.

When a healthy woman with a normal pregnancy is empowered to spontaneously labour without an epidural, nearly all give birth naturally, devoid of complications – that's a fact that has *oftentimes* gotten lost on busy hospital delivery units with staff who haven't *routinely* attended birth-centre or home-birth labours for a long time, if ever. It is easy to lose site of the fact that so many women give birth uneventfully.

It is well known that the routine early-administering of epidurals changes labour from "low-risk" to "high-risk" (thus, the consequential need for continuous fetal monitoring). Epidurals directly impact rates of the three leading causes of emergency C-sections: *Failure to dilatate* effectively; *obstructed descents*; and *fetal distress*. Whereas with healthy, normal pregnancies spontaneously going into labour at term who avoid epidurals, all three of these obstetric complications become relatively rare events.

As an interesting aside, some years ago, a retrospective study was done in South Auckland, New Zealand, that looked at the births of over 4000 low-risk pregnancies.

For the women who chose to labour in one of the three small local Birth Centres (rather than going to the major local hospital), they ended up statistically four times less likely to have an emergency C-section; 1½ times less likely to haemorrhage; and five times less likely to be admitted to the High Dependency / Intensive Care unit or an operating theatre. Plus, their newborns were three times less likely to have low APGAR scores, and half as likely to need admission to the Neonatal Unit.

The study's conclusion was that the main contributing reason for the dramatically worse outcome statistics at the major hospital was because at the birth centres these women *deliberately limited their own access to epidurals*, and instead they "surrendered" to the pain of natural labour, and consequently gave birth normally.

Some other asides of personal commentary:

In my study years as a student midwife, I never actually witnessed a primip epidural labour that concluded in a normal, unassisted birth.

In my years as a midwife, I've heard *many* women remark with regret they wish they had declined the epidural because "after that point everything went wrong" with their birth plan (which routinely would conclude as an emergency obstetric delivery).

In my years as a midwife, I've never heard a woman remark "I wish I'd had an epidural instead of giving birth naturally". Women rarely, if ever, feel that way!

"Frankly it really does not amaze me how expectant women will take charge of the naturopathic holistic health of themselves and their unborn babe, while mostly intentionally not discussing their decisions with their mainstream maternity health professional ... because that is exactly what I did too ... not telling my midwife/doctor about the medical herbs my naturopath was prescribing me. Not surprisingly my births were incredibly efficient.

"So why don't we as pregnant women tell our 'secret'?

"In my case, it was because I didn't want a biomedical person voicing their uneducated opinion on an alternative complementary therapeutic discipline, which I knew they were not formally trained in.

"I frankly was not interested in their opinion!

"I was in charge of my own and my baby's wellbeing, and always would be for years to come."

— Editor, Kathy Fray
IMHC Research e-Journal, 22 September 2019

Acknowledgements

There are five thank yous in particular I want to mention.

First, Helen Ellis (my sister), who was the conference manager for our first ever local inaugural symposium. I will forever be grateful for your belief in me. We did the whole thing on faith.

Second, Caroline Jack (of Events by Caro), who has been my personal godsend in helping me to manage our ongoing conferences – even through a global pandemic.

Third, our whanau (Māori for family) who accept me warts-and-all, *especially* our three grown children who make sure I keep it real. Love you to the moon and back! xxx

Fourth, our many close friends who are just all amaze-balls – especially all my gal-pals. Whether it's the deck or the dinner table, I'm soooo in my happy place with you all.

Finally, my husband, Mark, who for over 35 years has patiently tolerated and supported all my (sometimes crazy, often radical) "flights of fancy" – never questioning if I am doing the right thing for me, or for us. Thanks, babe, for always being by my BFF and Rock of Gibraltar!

About the Author

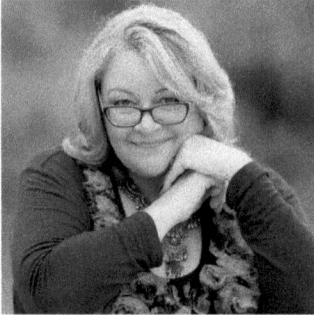

Kathy Fray is a semi-retired senior midwife who was trained in New Zealand (a country renowned for having one of the best maternity healthcare systems on the planet).

Kathy has been her country's number one best-selling birth/babies/motherhood author since 2005, and today is also managing director for the www.motherswise.com resources and services, creators of the world's No.1 online prenatal educational curriculum.

Kathy's other role is as the founding director for www.iimhco.com (International Integrative Maternity HealthCare Organization), who are global thought-leaders on *perinatal integrative medicine* (holistic maternal/fetal/neonatal wellness).

Today Kathy and her husband of more than three decades split their time between living in New Zealand's largest city, Auckland, and retreating to a waterfront home in remote Northland, NZ – and travelling internationally to attend conferences.

Kathy describes herself as a "work in progress".

www.KathyFray.com

www.MothersWise.com

www.IIMHCO.com

A healthy woman with a normal pregnancy; going spontaneously into labour at term; with a soft ripe cervix; with an empowered childbirth-educated mindset; with a non-anxious support crew; and with a holistic midwife or non-medicalized obstetrician; truly possesses the winning formula for her baby to experience a non-traumatic, non-dramatic, normal birth.

And if, under those circumstances, obstetric intervention is required, then everyone – woman, partner, midwife, obstetrician – can put their hands on their hearts and say 'We know we gave this baby's labour its best chance to conclude as a non-emergency delivery'.

Kathy Fray, Founding Director, IIMHCO

Other books by Kathy Fray

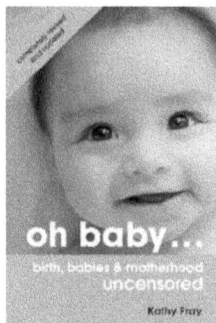

Oh Baby ... Birth, Babies & Motherhood Uncensored

A Penguin Random best-selling book since 2005, this is every mother-to-be's "Bible" that holds their hand, like a loving aunty ... from heavily pregnant through to their baby's first birthday, and everything in-between.

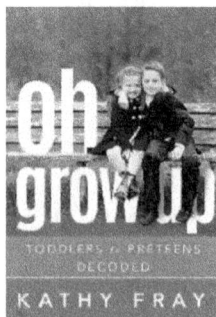

Oh Grow Up: Toddlers to Preteens Decoded

Kathy's popular sequel to Oh Baby ..., teaching "wholistic triadic" parenting: parenting their body using physiological IQ, parenting their mind using intellectual IQ, and parenting their spirit using soulful IQ.

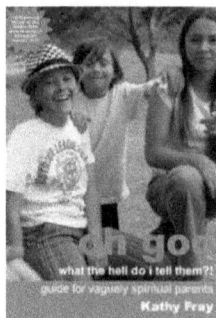

Oh God: What the Hell Do I Tell Them?! Guide for Vaguely Spiritual Parents

First runner-up winner at prestigious body-mind-spirit book awards, Kathy describes this book as being for the "hard core" of parents who want to equip their alpha Gen-Zs with old-age New Age cosmopolitan IQs no one ever taught us.

www.ingramcontent.com/pod-product-compliance
Lightning Source LLC
Chambersburg PA
CBHW060031030426
42334CB00019B/2276